Opening your Chakras:

A complete guide to finding balance by awakening, clearing & healing your chakras - For beginners & advanced practice in Reiki (2 in 1)

Siya Ishani

Table of Contents

Manuscript 1: Chakra Healing

Chapter 1 - Nothing Seems to Work for Me

Chapter 2- What Is NOT The Solution

Chapter 3 - Ailment Associations and A Brief History of Chakra Points

Chapter 4 - The 7 Basic Chakra Points

Chapter 5 - Development of the Chakras

Chapter 6 - Chakra Dissonance and Healing

Chapter 7 - Miscellaneous Chakra Exercises and More.

Chapter 8 - Kundalini energy - Historical background and understanding Kundalini

Chapter 9 - Preparations and steps for Releasing your Serpent Power

Chapter 10 - Kundalini Meditations and Exercises

Chapter 11- The Third Eye: Understanding and Opening your Sixth Sense

Chapter 12 - Energy Healing with Crystals and Other Stones

Chapter 13 - Chakra Meditation Garden

Chapter 14 - Kundalini and other Yoga forms

Conclusion

Manuscript 2: Reiki Healing

Introduction

Chapter 1 - Why try our approach to Reiki Healing?

Chapter 2 - Reiki History Primer

Chapter 3 - Reiki Basics - The Principles, How it works, and Meridians

Chapter 4 - Reiki Self-Healing Exercises

Chapter 5 - The Three Pillars and Reiki Healing for Others

Chapter 6 - Chakra points and Reiki: Are they compatible?

Chapter 7 - Incorporating Chakra Points into Reiki Healing

Chapter 8 - Reiki and Kundalini: Are they compatible?

Chapter 9 - Using Reiki in conjunction with Kundalini

Chapter 10 - Reiki - Full 12 Meridian Healing

Chapter 11 - Healing stones to incorporate into Reiki and Chakra Healings

Conclusion

Manuscript 1

Chakra Healing: A Practical Beginners Guide to Self-Healing.

Unblock, Awaken and Balance your Chakras. Open your Third Eye through Energy Healing and ancient Kundalini methods

Siya Ishani

© Copyright 2019 - All rights reserved.

The content contained within this book may not be reproduced, duplicated or transmitted without direct written permission from the author or the publisher.

Under no circumstances will any blame or legal responsibility be held against the publisher, or author, for any damages, reparation, or monetary loss due to the information contained within this book. Either directly or indirectly.

Legal Notice:

This book is copyright protected. This book is only for personal use. You cannot amend, distribute, sell, use, quote or paraphrase any part, or the content within this book, without the consent of the author or publisher.

Disclaimer Notice:

Please note the information contained within this document is for educational and entertainment purposes only. All effort has been executed to present accurate, up to date, and reliable, complete information. No warranties of any kind are declared or implied. Readers acknowledge that the author is not engaging in the rendering of legal, financial, medical or professional advice. The content within this book has been derived from various sources. Please consult a licensed professional before attempting any techniques outlined in this book.

By reading this document, the reader agrees that under no circumstances is the author responsible for any losses, direct or indirect, which are incurred as a result of the use of information contained within this document, including, but not limited to, — errors, omissions, or inaccuracies.

Table Of Contents

Table Of Contents

Chapter 1 - Nothing Seems To Work For Me

Chapter 2 - What Is NOT The Solution

Chapter 3 - Ailment Associations and A Brief History of Chakra Points

Chapter 4 - The 7 Basic Chakra Points

Chapter 5 - Development of the Chakras

Chapter 6 - Chakra Dissonance and Healing

Chapter 7 - Miscellaneous Chakra Exercises and More.

Chapter 8 - Kundalini energy - Historical background and understanding Kundalini

Chapter 9 - Preparations and steps for Releasing your Serpent Power

Chapter 10 - Kundalini Meditations and Exercises

Chapter 11 - The Third Eye: Understanding and Opening your Sixth Sense

Chapter 12 - Energy Healing with Crystals and Other Stones

Chapter 13 - Chakra Meditation Garden

Chapter 14 - Kundalini and other Yoga forms

Conclusion

Introduction

Between the years 1500 - 500 B.C. a series of Hindu scriptures known as the Vedas were written. They contained such lore as hymns, philosophies, and most importantly, guidance that could be followed in many aspects of life. Most importantly, parts of the texts described the ancient understanding of energy distribution in the body, known as Chakra points, as well as primal energy located in the base of the spine, known as Kundalini.

While skeptics abound, these writings have stood the test of time, drawing practitioners constantly over a span of more than 5000 years. How does this help you? Well, we are glad that you've asked. Manipulation of these energies can accomplish a number of things and we'll discuss them shortly in chapter 1. Of course, as the reader, feel free to skip ahead as you like if there are portions that you don't feel apply to you or that you are already familiar with. Our intent here is to provide a foundation in the basics of Chakra Points and Kundalini, Energy healing so that you can understand the vast scope of applications to which you can apply these energies.

Let's continue to chapter 1 and discuss some of what you may hope to accomplish with this ancient wisdom that has weathered the ages.

Chapter 1 - Nothing Seems to Work for Me

Though psychology, neurology, and other medical sciences have had amazing advances over time, it still seems that there is so much that is missed or misdiagnosed. Many of us suffer from a number of baneful habits and physical ailments that, try as we might, we can never seem to get to the root of them. As a result, at the very best we suffer unhappiness and at the worst, find ourselves dependent on band-aid style chemical solutions, prescribed and otherwise, that tend to help briefly with one or two symptoms while creating a dozen more. This is one of the most valid reasons why so many people are turning to Vedic wisdom with more than 3000 years of success as opposed to the younger, 'modern' sciences.

Some common examples of our collective suffering where this wisdom is being applied are as follows:

1. **Financial problems**- No matter how much money you make or how many budgets that you put together, you can never seem to save money. Living from paycheck to paycheck, there never seems to be enough, when logic tells you that there SHOULD be.

2. **Unhappiness with your Career**- You never seem to get promoted. Perhaps you aspire to a different career but can't bring yourself to take the leap. Work is simply work, something to do until you retire, unhappy.

3. **Discontentedness with your body**- You feel too fat or too thin. Unattractive. You find yourself going through fad diets or exercise regimens and the results are less than inspiring. Despite the medical viability of such options, calories consumed or denied,

you can't seem to achieve the physical form that you know lies there like a diamond in the rough.

4. **You don't feel that you can be loved**- Despite all your qualities, you find yourself shunning relationships or commitments because deep down, you have convinced yourself that you cannot be loved.

5. **You have difficulty with intimacy of the body and mind**- Get close to someone? No way! You find it impossible to let other people in. As a result, people only see a carefully cultivated image of you. Something shallow that you've cooked up to keep people at a distance and despite the desire to open up, for you it's simply not an option.

6. **Feeling powerless to achieve your dreams**- You have dreams and plans that never make it off of the drawing board, even though you know that if you could summon the energy to put into making these things happen that you would enjoy the success that would come of it. Yet you can't muster the energy for more than dreaming.

7. **Allergies the doctor cannot seem to diagnose**- You seem to be allergic to a number of things, yet the Doctor visits amount to little more than blanket antihistamines that make you feel more tired rather than well.

8. **You agree with others to avoid upsetting them**- Even when you know better, rather than 'rock the boat' you find yourself agreeing with others. This leads to immense stress and frustration in your life that you would gladly do away with... but no matter how you try you just can't seem to speak up.

9. **You can't seem to trust your intuition (even when it's always right.)**- This is a big one for many. No matter how many times your intuition has proven to be correct, you just can't bring yourself to trust it. This leads to missed opportunities in work, relationships, and life in general. You know this logically, why can't you trust yourself?

10. **You suffer from Migraines and stress headaches** - Chronic headaches are your constant companion, even when everything in life is going well and you aren't stressed at all. The Doctor doesn't know why. Psychology and Psychiatry have failed to give you a valid reason for this, yet it persists and there seems like no escape.

11. **Feeling disconnected from the spiritual**- Unable to get close to nature or the religion of your choice? Does the world around you feel more material than anything else, a machine rather than a collective of various energies and emotions? Has life become a matter of simply work, sleep, rinse and repeat? Many suffer from this and can't seem to find the reason why. We might have some help for you there.

12. **Chronic sore throat**- As soon as it's damp or cold, or even on a fair day, do you find yourself getting a sore or blocked-up feeling throat? Perhaps you are more susceptible to strep throat and there seems to be no medical reason why.

These are all common ailments and yet there seems to be nothing that anyone can do. So why don't the standard solutions seem to work? We understand the conundrum. To demonstrate this, let's discuss some of these same points in chapter 2 to better understand the solutions that were tried and the frustrating results that came instead of a solution. After we have demonstrated that we know and understand your frustrations, we'll let you in on OUR solution for these problems.

It's well worth the wait.

Chapter 2- What Is NOT The Solution

In the previous chapter we provided a list of common ailments. Many people experience them and many people try the same things, over and over, which are recommended by friends or physicians. Sadly, the results are always less than optimal. Stick with us and we will tell you why.

To show that we know what we're talking about, here is the list from Chapter 1 and some examples of things that you and many others have tried before deciding to look into the Vedic way of doing things.

Once we've discussed what you have tried we're going to let you in on a few secrets, things that you haven't tried, but that you will be glad of once you have. So here again, our list of ailments now appended with their commonly recommended "solutions".

1. Financial problems

Attempted solutions:

- Direct deposit into a second account, but instead of saving you just use the second card to withdraw impulsively.
- Budget after budget; You've kept track for a few days but something always comes up and you stop tracking or simply track your failures.
- Hiring an Accountant, resulting in 'sorry, I spent it' conversations.

Results: Financial instability is a vicious cycle. It results in frustration, missed opportunities, and embarrassment when around your friends and colleagues who wonder why you can't join them for lunch or the occasional outing. It can prevent you from owning a home rather than renting one or building a nest-egg to supplement your retirement. It's a serious problem indeed.

2. Unhappiness with your Career

Attempted solutions:

- Constant training at your current job that never gets used.
- Job-hopping with no idea where you want to be.
- Expensive college courses with no direction.
- Starting your own business before you might be ready.

Results: Unhappiness with your chosen career path can be devastating. It can affect your morale and your inner-compass, after all, if you don't know what you wish to aspire to in your career, how can you steer the rest of your life? If the solutions above haven't helped in the slightest, there is likely another sort of imbalance at play that you were not aware of. We'll explain it to you very soon.

3. Discontentedness with your body

Attempted solutions:

- Any number of Fad diets, many of which leave you light headed and famished all of the time and are unsustainable in the long run.
- Gym memberships that never get used.
- Personal trainers that leave you exhausted with little results.
- Attending Support groups with people that you can't even relate to in the slightest.

Results: This is a big one. How can you be happy with life if you aren't happy with the person that you see in the mirror? Worse, failure to achieve your goals when you are suffering so much can lead to a complete lack of energy, resulting in reclusiveness and laziness in the overall ennui encompassing you, which makes the problem worse. The nail in the coffin is when the Doctor can't find any reasons wrong or when they give you blanket excuses that you know are simply not true or don't apply to you. You'll be glad to know that there is another way.

4. You don't feel that you can be loved

Attempted solutions:

- Spending time with potential mates that are shallow and thus 'safe'.
- Rushing into physical intimacy before you are ready.
- Becoming a recluse to avoid the issue altogether.
- Devoting too much time to work and hobbies to 'keep busy'

Results: Numerous bad things can result from this. Reliance on alcohol or drugs. Ill-conceived 'flings' for a quick, emotional rush that never lasts. Seclusion that blunts your social skills more, making it harder to make a connection in the future should you feel ready. There is a reason for this that is 'behind the scenes' and we will tell you what it is in our next chapter, so that you may empower yourself to defeat this debilitating affliction.

5. You have difficulty with intimacy of the body and mind

Attempted Solutions:

- Seeking the company of people, you know engender no emotional or physical responses in you.
- Psychologist sessions or Psychiatrist chemical cocktails for a diagnosed 'condition' you feel that you probably don't really have.

- You force yourself into attempted intimacy that you are not yet ready for.

Results: Unhappy relationships, feelings of being misunderstood, fear that your heart is simply 'cold'. Misplaced anger can result when meeting or speaking with others who do not suffer from this issue. This is a great source of unhappiness and can seriously damage your self-image. Thankfully, there is a Vedic aspect to this issue that we will teach you that can make a huge difference and help you to interact with confidence and honesty that resonate deeply within yourself.

6. Feeling powerless to achieve your dreams

Attempted solutions:

- Constantly reading biographies of those who have achieved success in the hopes of inspiration that won't be acted upon.
- Endless plan-outlining in notebooks without embarking on any steps
- Spending money on career-coaching or entrepreneur courses without using what you've learned.

Results: You find yourself forced into feeling like a dilettante, a dabbler, a daydreamer, accomplishing nothing but always plotting and planning. This leads to feeling effete and ineffectual. Worse, often the planning is good, resulting in 'friends' stealing your ideas and the subsequent success that could have come with them. There are other ways to energize your goal-drive and lead yourself to success. We will discuss this thoroughly in the next chapter.

7. Allergies the doctor cannot seem to diagnose

Attempted solutions:

- Trying over the counter antihistamines, often mixing them in combinations that are not necessarily recommended.
- Endless doctor visits.
- Alternative therapies, such as acupuncture, dietary changes, and other more holistic approaches that are still proving ineffective.

Results: Unexplained allergies can be a source of a number of frustrations. They can make you a social pariah. You might be viewed by others or by yourself as 'weak'. Constant drowsiness or hyper alertness can result from antihistamine overuse or from mixing over the counter drugs in an attempt to find relief. What many do not realize, however, is that bodily responses such as this are not always medical in nature. They are symptoms, yes, but not of what you might think. We'll discuss this further.

8. You agree with others to avoid upsetting them

Attempted solutions:

- Self-esteem books or courses.
- Avoiding meetings with dominant personalities
- Overcompensating in physical or mental training in an attempt to raise morale.

Results: Typically anger and self-loathing can come from this sort of scenario. Your opinions are just as valid, if not more so in some cases, than others who are pushing you around. Worse, some personality types notice your reluctance to disagree and may use this to support their own agendas. The self-esteem required to speak-up is actually associated with a particular Chakra that we will teach you about and you may just find in it that edge that you've been needing all this time.

9. You can't seem to trust your intuition (even when it's always right.)

Attempted solutions:

- Psychology sessions to determine why you don't trust yourself.
- 'Intuition journals' that reaffirm that you should trust your intuition but still prove ineffectual.
- Taking unhealthy gambles or actually gambling in an effort to encourage self-trust.

Results: Failure to trust your gut-instinct can result in the frustration of missed connections, lost adventure possibilities, being passed for job promotions, and more. While you don't want to base every decision on a whim, learning to trust your intuition is important in this journey that we call life. You can learn the right times to trust your intuition, however, with the right knowledge. We'll be happy to share it with you.

10. You suffer from Migraines and stress headaches

Attempted solutions:

- Over the counter and prescription medications (often sporting awful side-effects or over-reliance)
- Numerous fruitless doctor visits
- Psychiatry visits to rule out stress, resulting in further medications that you don't really need and side-effects of their own.

Results: Migraines and stress headaches can be horribly debilitating, resulting in loss of work and leisure time, and as such we will often overmedicate ourselves and still lose these things, trading our pain for drowsiness and dozens of side-effects. There is also a huge frustration when we receive diagnosis after diagnosis that feel more like excuses than something that might actually apply to us. Sometimes the answer isn't something that you'll find in a medical practitioner's guide, but in a much older series of texts.

11. Feeling disconnected from the spiritual

Attempted solutions:

- Overcompensating attempting to force a spiritual experience.
- Gravitation to various religious groups in hope of 'finding yourself' and touch your spiritual side again.
- Taking an Atheistic approach and denying your own and other's spirituality completely

Results: *We are spiritual creatures by nature. Think of it from a scientific approach. The superstrings theory at its basics states that all matter is energy vibrating at a certain wavelength. We also know that all energy has to go somewhere. Without even invoking deities or specific religions we have, at the core, a relationship with all things around us by the very nature of our existence. Energy doesn't have to be denominational. Denial of our natural state of existence can lead to general unhappiness, feelings of being uninspired, and can make us feel that we are not a part of the great whole that is around us. Thankfully, understanding of Chakras and Kundalini is an understanding of energies. You might be surprised at the transformation in your views on spirituality that can come with this.*

12. Chronic sore throat

Attempted solutions:

- Daily rituals such as gargling salt water(yuck!)
- Constant Doctor visits
- Prohibitive quantities of antibiotics each year

Results: *This is an ailment suffered by many and Doctors end up telling us 'you're just very susceptible to sore throat.' As such, this* results in an enormous amount of physical suffering and loss of time at work or in leisure paying visit after visit to the doctor or the local pharmacy for over-the-counter lozenges. It eats up your sick days at work and can make it difficult when public speaking is required or when you want to socialize. The good news is that this is not necessarily a strictly-medical condition.

Now that we've got your attention it's time to get to the fun part:

Chakras

In the following chapter we will discuss the benefits that the Vedic wisdom of Chakra energy can bring into your life for mitigation or, in some cases, complete removal of these ailments and more.

We'll follow it with a brief history in regards to Chakra points as well in order to show to you how long that others just like you have been employing this ancient wisdom to succeed where the advice of well-meaning friends and physicians have failed.

Chapter 3 - Ailment Associations and A Brief History of Chakra Points

Now that we have established a list of sample problems that many of us face today, we are going to begin this chapter with some of the benefits that may be realized by learning and strengthening various Chakra points by highlighting their correlations from the ailments list that we provided in the previous chapters. After that, we intend to illuminate the history of Chakra points for you so that you will have a little background into this most ancient of sciences. From there, we will proceed to the next chapter where we will give you details on each individual Chakra point and then begin building your knowledge on how to strengthen and balance each. Sound good? Let's proceed.

So, to begin, here is a list of the 7 Chakra points, along with the 12 sample ailments which we listed in the previous chapters, listed by association with their governing Chakra point.

Empowering these Chakra points can help you to balance the Chakra energies in order to correct these issues (and more, which we will discuss in Chapter 4 'The 7 basic Chakra points').

So, without further ado, here is our updated list:

1st Chakra - Root Chakra

- Financial Problems.
- Unhappiness with your career.

- Discontentedness with your body.
- You don't feel that you can be loved.

2nd Chakra - Sacral Chakra

- You have difficulty with intimacy of the body and mind.

3rd Chakra - Solar Plexus Chakra

- Feeling powerless to achieve your dreams.

4th Chakra - Heart Chakra

- Allergies the doctor cannot seem to diagnose.

5th Chakra - Throat Chakra

- You agree with others to avoid upsetting them.
- Chronic sore throat.

6th Chakra - Third Eye Chakra

- You can't seem to trust your intuition.

7th Chakra - Crown Chakra

- You suffer from Migraines and stress headaches.
- Feeling disconnected from the spiritual.

Intrigued? The sampling which we've given in progression through these chapters is just a taste of what understanding and mastery of these energies can bring into your life. People worldwide have been using this system for over 3000 years, after all. We're going to go into that history next so that you have a little grounding on the foundations of Chakra points. Once we have paved a little solid footing for you to start we will go into detail in the following chapters on the 7 basic Chakra points and exercises to build and empower them to utilize to your own advantage.

So, Chakra points... What's that all about?

In India, circa 1000-1500 B.C. (this is the general consensus, though there is some contention) the Vedic texts were written. Concerning hymns, traditions, prayers, poems, philosophies, and more, these texts encompassed the tenets and basics of the Vedic religion. This is where we first have written mention of the Chakras. They are essentially the recorded oral tradition of the Brahmans, the Priests, highest of the social caste in India. Due to their education, these priests often acted in advisory and ministerial capacities to warriors and ruling chiefs.

The first mention of Chakras of which we have written account originated here. The word 'Chakra', literally means wheel, and referred to the chariot wheels of the rulers. Visualized as a spinning wheel of light, there are also associations with the sun. The first mentions that we have of the Chakras as spiritual centers of energy came about in 600 B.C.E. in the Yoga Upanishads, another Sanskrit text dealing with Yogic traditions. Lore of the Chakras would not actually come to the west in printed form until 1919, when an Englishman named Arthur Avalon published a translation of texts from 1577(entitled 'Sat-Cakra-Nirupana') and the 10th century (A text entitled 'Padaka-Pancaka' and another called 'Gorakshashatakam'). These texts contained information of the Chakra centers as well as instructions on meditating upon these centers to empower the self. Needless to say, the ancient lore was well-received and with the floodgates open, more and more information about this system began to flood into the West.

The rest is, well, history.

So, what exactly are Chakra points?

Chakra points are simply energy centers. While the majority of focus is on 7 main Chakras (and that is what we will focus on, as this is meant to be an introductory text), there are actually 114 Chakra points with 72,000 nadis (energy channels) through which Prana, or 'vital energy', travels.

The 7 Chakra points on which we will focus on in this book, interestingly enough, correspond, top to bottom, with the 7 main nerve ganglia of the spinal column. While visualized as a halo-type wheel of light, these correspondences will help you to better understand how the Chakra points map in your own body. We'll discuss corresponding locations in further detail in Chapter 4.

Now, these energy points govern various 'spheres' of influence in your life. The balances of your overall life-energy. Understanding of these Chakra points can help you to see when particular aspects of your energies are blocked or oversaturated. This can help you to achieve a balance, empowering yourself where it's needed, leading to a better enjoyment of life and banishment of the elements of discord that blockage can introduce into your life.

Sounds a little complicated, no?

Don't worry. Our job here is to give you a basic grounding in the lore that you can apply and build upon. A foundation, if you will. In this magnificent age of information, a little Google time and some recreational reading on your phone, E-book reader, or library of your choice can get you the nitty-gritty on some of the more complicated concepts. Here we will focus on getting you started and giving you the skills to GET RESULTS and the rest is up to you. Once you have seen what the ancient wisdom can do for you then you will understand why so many people spend a lifetime increasing their understanding and mastery of their Chakras.

Now that we have given you a crash-course in the history as well as the general knowledge of what Chakra points are and some things that they can do for you, we think you are ready to dive a little deeper. In the next chapter we will identify the 7 Chakras in detail and give you a better understanding of their spheres of influence so that you know exactly what they can do for you. Once you know a little more about this system then a lot of things in your life are going to make more sense.

Count on it. Now, on to chapter 4, 'The 7 Basic Chakra Points'.

Chapter 4 - The 7 Basic Chakra Points

Now that we have gone into some grounding, let's discuss the 7 major Chakra points, their corresponding locations, and spheres of influence. First, the names and locations of the Chakras are as follows:

Sanskrit name and Translation: *Location:*
    Commonly called:

1. *Muladhara* "root or support"   Base of spine

Root Chakra

2. *Svadhishthana* "sweetness"   Below the navel

Sacral Chakra

3. *Manipura* "lustrous gem"   Stomach

Solar Plexus Chakra

4. *Anahata* "unstruck"   Central chest

Heart Chakra

5. *Vishuddha* "purification"   Throat base

Throat Chakra

6. *Ajna* "to perceive"   Forehead, center above eyes

Third Eye Chakra

7. *Sahasrara* "Thousandfold"   Top of the head

Crown Chakra

As mentioned previously, the Chakras are most commonly visualized as circles of light, but it's easiest to remember as a beginner by thinking of a straight line of points going up your spine.

Next we want to describe to you their spheres of influence so that you have a better idea of the energies that they govern. Later in this book we will discuss symptoms of blockage of these particular Chakras, so that you can zero in on problems as you find them to obtain a more balanced energy in life.

Here is our list of the basic influence areas of the 7 Chakras:

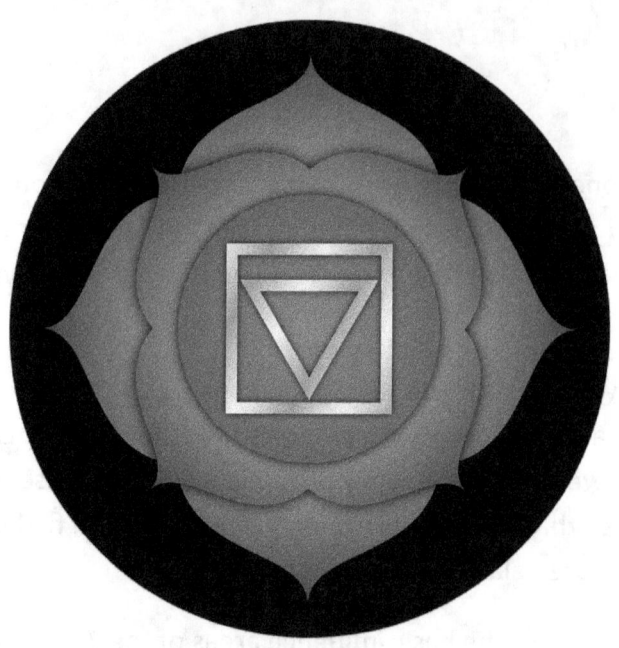

1. Root Chakra

- Influence in Life: The root chakra rules over areas such as survival/self preservation, material aspects of life, as well as sexuality as it relates to procreation in a security aspect, predominantly survival and procreation. Largely tied with your ability to feel safe and secure, the Root Chakra also governs your fight or flight reflexes. Think of this as the self-security Chakra or perhaps more accurately, self-preservation.
- Physical Associations: This Chakra associates with the male sexual organs, Coccyx, Legs, hips, and the lower back

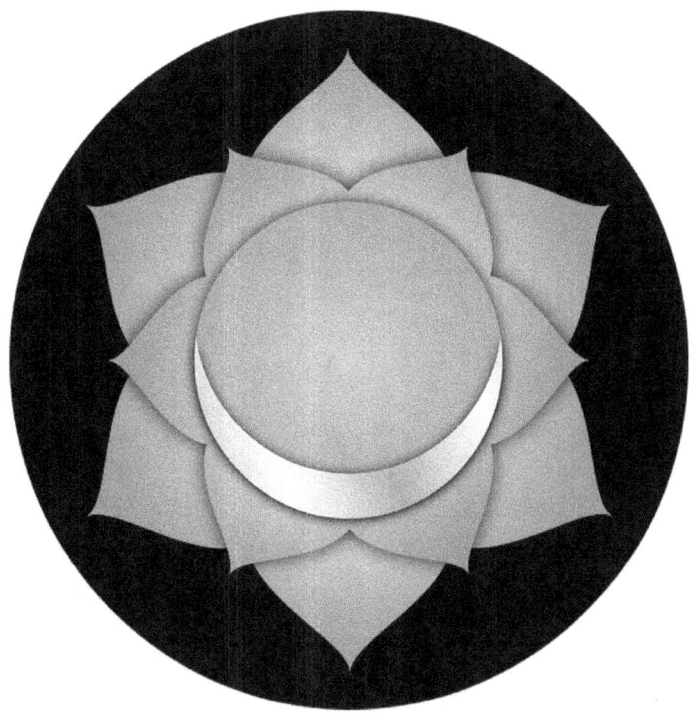

2. Sacral Chakra

- Influence in Life: The Sacral Chakra is associated emotionally with how we connect with others and experiences in life. Family, friends, sexual partners, and general experiences... Yes, experiences. How you feel when you view a sunrise or witness the birth of your child. This Chakra is tied to such things. It's also associated strongly with the sense of self and how we broadcast to others. How much you let yourself feel and also utilize your self-power. Thus it governs your inner strength as well as how you share that strength with others.
- Physical Associations: Female sexual organs, bladder, colon, and the large intestine.

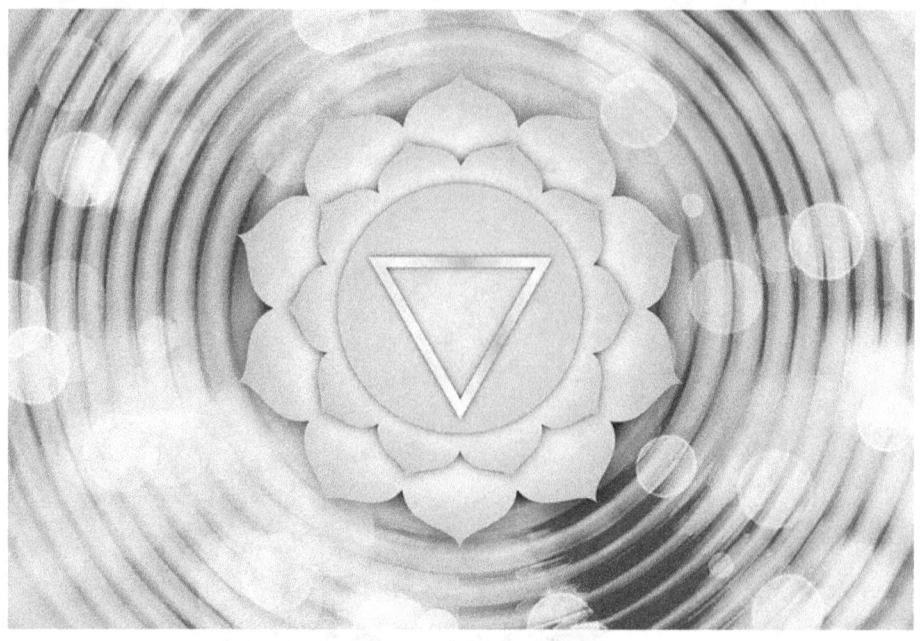

3. Solar Plexus Chakra

- Influence in Life: While the Sacral Chakra defines how you utilize your self-power; the Solar Plexus Chakra is essentially the seat of said power. It defines self-acceptance, as well as the ability to recognize and understand who you truly are as well as your ability to accurately represent yourself to the world at large. This is strongly tied with your Professional and Personal life, as it relates to personal abilities, and affects your ability to feel pride and self-worth.
- Physical Associations: The Solar Plexus Chakra governs the kidneys, gall bladder, stomach, liver, and the pancreas.

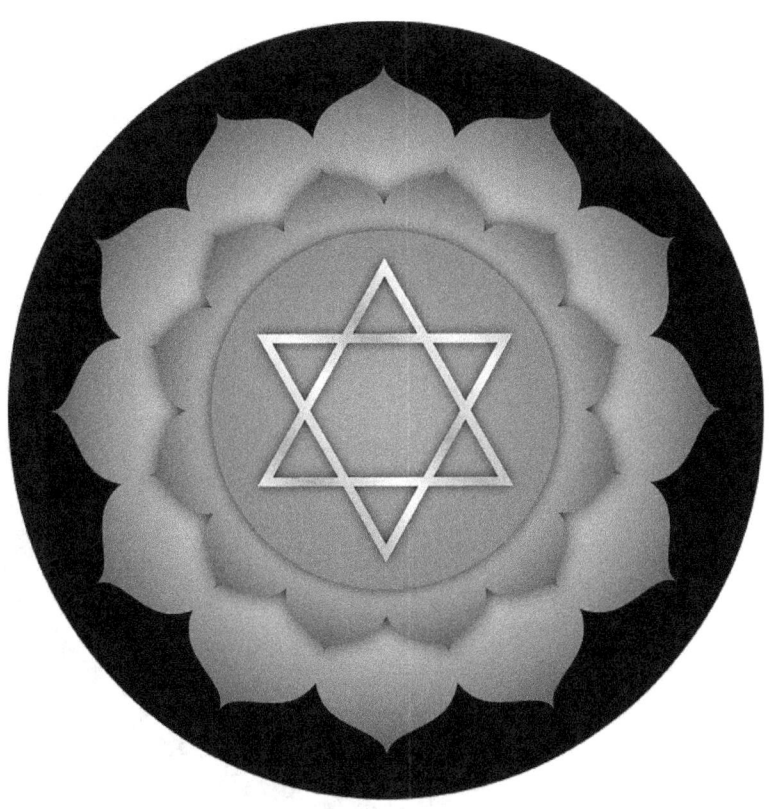

4. Heart Chakra

- Influence in Life: The Heart Chakra holds influence on the ability to love, both for the self and with others. It also affects how we interpret experiences and lessons in life, as such wisdom is always filtered by that variable of 'do I love myself?'. In this capacity, it's the difference between learning a life's lesson or deciding the world is against you.
- Physical Associations: This Chakra governs the heart, upper back, lungs, breasts, arms, and the lungs.

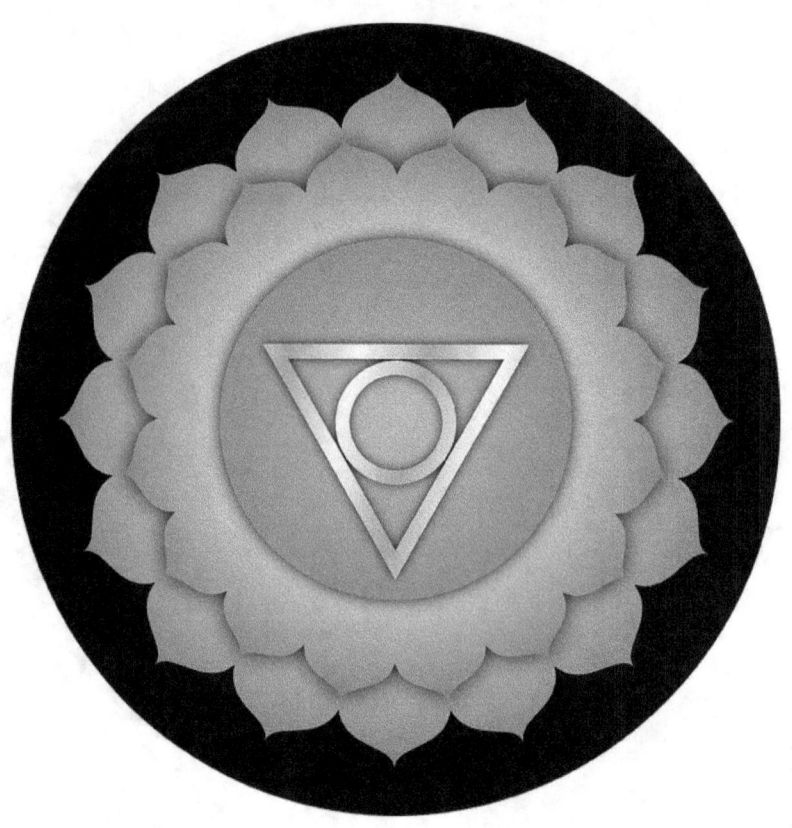

5. Throat Chakra

- Influence in Life: The Throat Chakra governs communication, both with others as well as with the self. As such, it's also strongly associated with the ability to express one's creativity. This also affects your ability to express dreams or ideas in a 'concrete' way so that the rest of the world might see and understand.
- Physical Associations: The Throat Chakra encompasses the areas of the neck, throat, mouth, ears, thyroid, and the larynx.

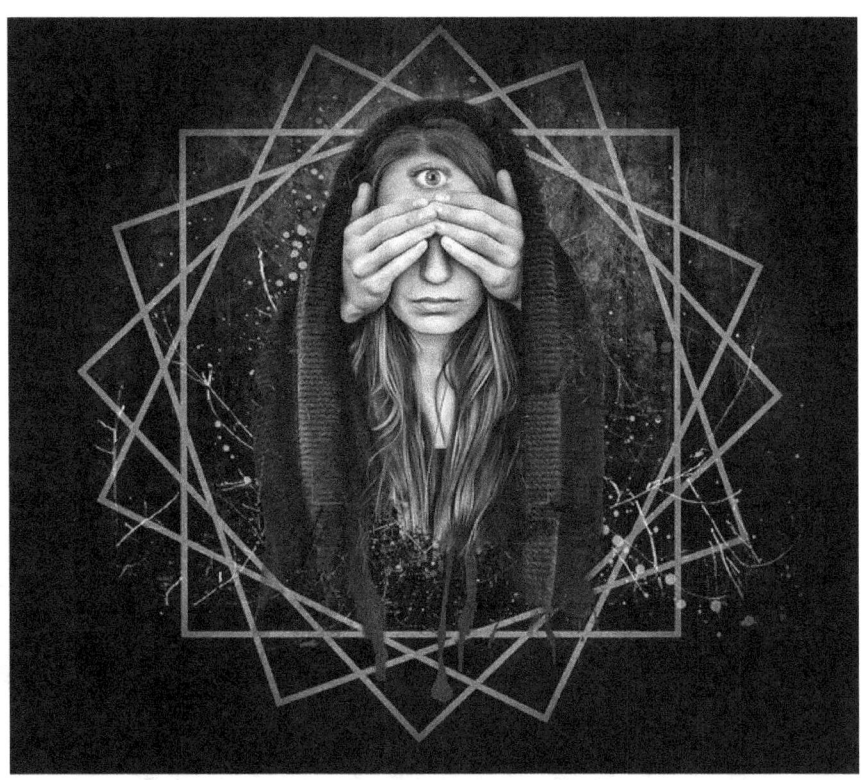

6. Third Eye Chakra

- Influence in Life: The Third Eye Chakra influences spiritual awareness as well as the ability to think logically and clearly. It lets you see the bigger picture, in both a material and spiritual manner. It also enables understanding of the true self.
- Physical Associations: This Chakra associates with the lymph nodes, brain, eyes, sinuses, endocrine system, and the pineal gland.

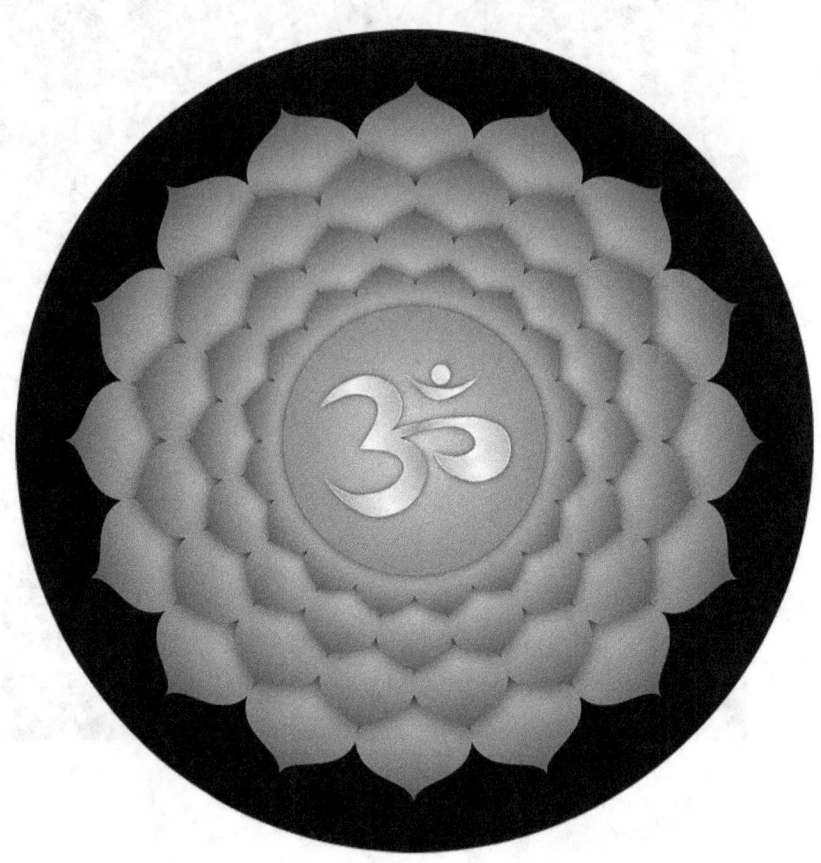

7. Crown Chakra

- Influence in Life: While the Third Eye Chakra governs spiritual awareness, the Crown Chakra is the seat of one's spiritual power. It governs the connection of the self with the spiritual realms or aspects of life around you. It contributes to one's view of connectedness with the universe and helps to provide a stronger awareness of the future to come.
- Physical Associations: The Crown Chakra is associated with the cervical vertebrae, the spine, and the joints.

Now that we have established the locations and primary functions of the 7 basic Chakra Points our next step is to discuss how one can develop these points. In Chapter 5 we will discuss the development of these Chakra points so that you can begin to utilize their power for yourself.

Are you ready? Good. Then let's proceed now then to the next chapter so that we can develop that Chakra energy and put it to good use. Rest assured that you will be quite pleased with the results.

Chapter 5 - Development of the Chakras

Development of the Chakras is something that anyone can do. It's quick and easy, rather, in that these are energy points in your body that are already there and active. You just need to learn to develop your focus and awareness. Awareness will also help you to know when one Chakra may be more active then another, so that you can take advantage of this or lessen its influence for more balanced energies as-needed. As we have mentioned before, your Chakras rules various portions of the body and the spirit. Learning about these energies can help you to achieve better health and a better piece of mind. The study of these can be as devoted or as simple as you like. A mild read every morning for a few weeks or a controlled study of a few days. That is all up to you. Let's get to the practical aspects.

So what is the easiest way to access these energies?

Meditation.

First, a simple breathing exercise is required. Proper breathing ensures that you will be in a relaxed and receptive state in which you can proceed to a deeper meditative one, blocking out all distractions so that you may focus on your Chakras. As your first breathing exercise, let's do a simple 3-3-3.

3-3-3 Breathing Exercise

The 3-3-3 breathing exercise is quite useful, in that it's simple, elegant, and effective. Seat yourself somewhere that you feel comfortable and close your eyes.

Bow, breathe in slowly for a count of three

One.

    Two.

        Three.

Next, Hold your breath for a slow count of three.

One.

    Two.

        Three.

Lastly, simply exhale slowly for a count of three

One.

    Two.

        Three.

Practice doing this in 10 minute intervals. Do you notice your heart slowing as you become more relaxed? The great thing about this exercise is that you can vary the counts for different results that you will discover on your own. Try flooding yourself with oxygen by doing a 4-3-3 breathing session, or lessening it slightly with a 3-4-3.

There are many possibilities, some that lessen pain or increase focus, and best of all, with practice your body will remember them and you will find yourself breathing automatically in certain patterns that you have discovered on your own in times of stress or duress (some have reported with this exercise that emergencies such as a car accident or other physically damaging trauma have automatically triggered a controlled breathing response, so be sure to practice your breathing.) Practice throughout the week to find your optimal combination or if you are already comfortable with the 3-3-3 to the point that you don't have the distraction of counting to derail your focus, then we are ready to proceed to the meditations.

Now that you've got a handle on proper breathing we can move on to some basic Chakra meditation.

So, what is Chakra meditation? With standard meditation we reach a relaxed state in which, devoid of thought, we become better aware of the self and the universe around us. Chakra meditation, however, involves achieving a meditative state in which we focus upon specific Chakra energies which, in turn, gives us a laser-focus on particular aspects of our physical and mental well-being as it relates to the Chakra point. These sorts of meditations can be a great means to achieve a better sense of well-being, both spiritually and physically, as you are soon to find out.

Let's begin with a simple meditation to increase our awareness of the Chakras.

First Meditation Exercise - Exploring your Chakras

Preparation:

- Find yourself a quiet place. Within the home where you are comfortable or if possible, a nearby forest or even your backyard where you can be close to nature.
- Be sure that you may be seated comfortably. A lotus position is nice and traditional, however, the focus here is on achieving a meditative state... on relaxing. This means that you can cheat tradition a little if you like. Sit on the couch or a comfortable camping chair if you are out in the woods.
- Keep in mind that this will take a half hour, possibly more if you find yourself in a particularly contemplative mood. That means you will want to make sure you've nothing scheduled for that time and that you have set your phone to 'silent'(not vibrate, coming suddenly out of a meditative state can be a jarring experience). This will ensure no interruptions, at least as much as is possible in this sometimes-chaotic world of ours.
- For your first few times, if you do not wish to memorize the steps, then make a recording of yourself reading the steps which you can listen to on your portable mp3 or other media player of your choice, so that you may follow the instructions more easily. If you opt for this method, be sure to leave pauses for a few minutes in between steps where you are asked to visualize something, so that as you sit there with your eyes closed, becoming more relaxed, you will find yourself with sufficient time to experience and sharpen your visualizations to the fullest.
- Note that for this meditation we will use different colors to represent the Chakra points., incorporating the 7 colors of the rainbow. Color schemes for various Chakras were something added much later, so while they are useful, please keep in mind that they are not necessarily as steeped in tradition as some of the other information that you are learning.
    - Crown Chakra – Red
    - Third Eye Charka – Orange
    - Throat Charka – Yellow

- Heart Charka – Green
- Solar Plexus Chakra – Blue
- Sacral Chakra – Indigo
- Root Chakra - Violet

Meditation steps:

1. If you are seated comfortably, begin breathing properly to get yourself relaxed.

2. Close your eyes.

3. Start by visualizing the top portion of your head, the Crown Chakra. Visualize a red light there and let your thoughts drain away to all but focus upon this light. Let it fill you, energize you… Feel it burning away the negative emotions; fear, anger, guilt, jealousy. Anything that is distracting you. Like logs being burned, let these negative emotions feed the light that you see in your mind. Notice how it gets brighter and brighter. When it's at its brightest and remains blazing, unchanged, then this Chakra is energized. It's time to move down to the Third Eye Chakra.

4. Feel the energy seeping down from your Crown Chakra to the space slightly above and between your eyes, the Third Eye Chakra. As it seeps down, see the Red energy becoming Orange at the Third Eye point, dripping there like water in trickles down your forehead at first until it becomes a steady flow. See the glow radiating from the Third Eye point. Like a radar depiction in movies, see the light expanding, pulsing out in a wide circumference, a three-dimensional sphere of bright orange light, so that it touches everything around you as it grows brighter and more powerful. Once it's at its brightest, we can move down to the Throat Chakra.

5. See the orange color rushing down from the powerful Third Eye to the point at the base of your throat, suffusing the Throat Chakra with a light that is rapidly transformed from orange to yellow. See if fill as is you are powering a small, yellow sun. Contemplate upon this tiny sun at your Throat Chakra until you are ready to send the energy once more down.

6. Send the energy of the tiny sun down to the center of your chest, to the Heart Chakra. Visualize the yellow energy becoming as a powerful light-green, such as you might see in nature in the beginning of Spring. Let the energy trickle slowly as the green light slowly grows. Once this emerald light is at it's brightest, let the energy drift down further, to the stomach, changing from green to a sapphire blue.

7. As the energy moves down to your stomach, the Solar Plexus Chakra, visualize it crackling into place like electricity, rendering itself frozen in place as it grows into deeper sapphire hues. Once this light is shining brightly and seems to be growing no further, let the energy drift crackle down to the spot just below your navel, the Sacral Chakra.

8. See the energy crackling as if into an empty glass sphere at your Sacral Chakra point. As it fills the sphere the energy changes color from blue to indigo (almost purple but closer to blue on the color wheel. Google can show you the exact hue). When the energy from your Solar Plexus Chakra as completely emptied into the Sacral Chakra, let the glass sphere change from glass into a light, expanding and brightening with your focus upon it. Contemplate this light for as long as you like, minutes or moments. When the intensity of the light becomes static, unchanging, then let the light flow in rivulets further down still to the base of your spine.

9. As the light reaches the base of your spine, the Root Chakra, see it changing color once again, shifting subtly to violet hues of light. Let this light grow stronger as it flows from the Sacral Chakra to the Root Chakra until all of the energy has been transferred. See it growing in intensity until the light is at it's fullest, as with the previous points, and hold your focus upon it in contemplation. Keep thoughts from your mind, only focus on the color and intensity of the light.

10. Now visualize all of the Chakras lighting up, from root to crown, blazing all with equal light. Once you can hold this vision in your mind and see it perfectly, slowly open your eyes. The exercise has ended.

Now that we have finished the first meditation there are a few things to ask yourself:

- Were any of the colors/Chakras brighter than the others to begin with in your visualizations?
- Were any of them dimmer or harder to empower?
- Did you notice any introspection that came randomly to you when you were meditating upon a particular Chakra point?

The reason for these questions is that dimmer colors in some areas can indicate blockage, stronger colors might indicate that we are unknowingly energizing a particular Chakra at the time. The introspection is important, as the Chakras not only govern particular thought patterns but correspond with particular parts of the body. With practice, you can modify this simple meditation to focus on a specific Chakra if you feel that there might be discord in order to give yourself a deeper understanding of what is at play with that particular Chakra. Blockage of a particular Chakra (or more than one) can and does occur, in the next chapter we will discuss this in detail in regards to symptoms that you can look for that might be an indication of Chakra-blockage as well as exercises that may be employed in the healing of such blockages. Until you are ready for this chapter, practice the meditation that we've just taught you. It's good to do it when you have time throughout the week to help get you to feeling balanced and energized.

Now that we have taught you the first meditation, let's proceed to Chapter 6 'Chakra Dissonance and Healing' so that you can learn the signs of Chakra blockage and exactly what to do about them.

Chapter 6 - Chakra Dissonance and Healing

In our previous chapter we taught you a basic method to get a glimpse of your Chakra points and to lightly energize them. Exercises such as these are useful when there is a Chakra imbalance as well, although there is quite a wide variety of things that you can do of which you might not be aware of. That's where we come in, of course.

So how do you know if your Chakras may be imbalanced? As it turns out, there are quite a few signs and symptoms that can indicate a Chakra Imbalance. In this chapter we are going to list each Chakra as well as detailed information regarding Physical, Mental, and Behavioral symptoms that can indicate a blockage of a particular Chakra that needs to be dealt with. Following this, we will list each Chakra again with information as to how you can combat the blockage of each of the Chakras.

Let's begin.

1. Root Chakra

Physical symptoms: Blockage of the Root Chakra can result in a number of issues. As it ties with feelings of security and well-being, blockage may result in issues with overeating. Other issues that can arise include kidney stones, constipation, prostate issues, sciatica, issues with the legs or knees, and even impotence.

Mental/Behavioral Symptoms: Blockage of this Chakra can result in feelings of paranoia, insecurity, general distrust, and sometimes result in 'wandering feet' due to the feeling that you are never quite home. You may feel abandoned at times. In relationships, codependency issues may arise.

2. Sacral Chakra

Physical symptoms: Like the Root Chakra, blockage of the Sacral Chakra can result in kidney problems. Beyond this, bladder problems can occur, as well as such issues as back pain, urinary tract infections, ovarian cysts, and even infertility.

Mental/Behavioral Symptoms: As this Chakra governs how you deal with people, broadcast yourself, and how you utilize your inner strength, blockage of this Chakra can be quite dangerous. You may find yourself developing a nasty temper, severe jealousy, or both. Sexually, a low or nonexistent libido, failure to achieve orgasms, or premature ejaculation can occur. Blockage can also cause one to become manipulative, obsessed with sex, or you might find yourself feeling completely out of control of your life.

3. Solar Plexus Chakra

Physical symptoms: Overall health is heavily associated with this Chakra. Such ailments as diabetes, digestive issues, ulcers, arthritis, fibromyalgia, asthma, liver, and gall bladder issues are associated with imbalance for this particular Chakra. This is definitely one to pay attention to.

Mental/Behavioral Symptoms: Blockage of this Chakra can be vicious, as this is the seat of the self. Disconnection from one's identity can occur, causing you to feel lost. Coping skills can be affected, causing slow or even NO healing in cases of trauma. You may find yourself being pushed into decisions that you don't agree with as people notice and take advantage of the loss of self. Another warning sign of a blocked Solar Plexus Chakra is a sudden failure in being able to set boundaries with others. Loss of self control, anxiety, and even addictions (physical and chemical) can become a problem when there is blockage present in this Chakra.

4. Heart Chakra

Physical symptoms: Respiratory issues such as asthma or allergies are associated with Heart Chakra issues. Other ailments, such as heart disease, hypertension, and poor circulation are also associated with this Chakra.

Mental/Behavioral Symptoms: Blockage of the Heart Chakra can result in feelings of loneliness, general distrust in friendships and relationships, even cruelty. Compassion and your ability to love are governed by this Chakra, you see, and thus your ability to feel love or understanding in regards to emotional issues your friends or your mate might be experiencing can result when there are problems with this Chakra. Social anxiety and suspicion of gifts or difficulty giving them can also occur, so watch for these signs, they may indicate that your Heart Chakra needs attention.

5. Throat Chakra

Physical symptoms: Blockage of the Throat Chakra can result in a number of issues. A chronic sore throat, ulcers of the mouth, laryngitis, frequent neck pain, thyroid issues, disorders of the jaw, and even problems with the teeth.

Mental/Behavioral Symptoms: Blockage can result in a massive drop in communication skills, resulting in failure to express yourself, shyness, social anxiety, and feelings of social detachment. In severe cases, the adverse can occur, and you may find yourself becoming unintentionally manipulative, domineering, deceptive, or even arrogant. Suddenly finding yourself always quiet in social situations can be a definitive sign of Throat Chakra blockage.

6. Third Eye Chakra

Physical symptoms: As the Third Eye Chakra associates strongly with your head and brain, issues with this Chakra may result in frequent headaches, eye pain, insomnia, and in serious cases, even seizures or serious delusions may occur. Poor vision suddenly occurring when your eyesight was fine before may also be a sign of an issue with the Third Eye Chakra. Vivid nightmares invading your sleep all of the sudden are also a warning sign so be sure not to ignore this, it means that your Third Eye Chakra needs attention.

Mental/Behavioral Symptoms: Blockage of this Chakra can lead to a loss of direction in life as you stop trusting your inner voice. You may find yourself suddenly obsessed with the past or completely disinterested in your own future. Forgoing your intuition can lead to you guiding yourself through selective memories and deception may occur in order to hide your lack of foresight.

7. Crown Chakra

Physical symptoms: Neurological problems, Depression, Migraine headaches, and nerve pain are associated with this Chakra. Thyroid and Pineal gland issues are also associated with blockage of this Chakra. In the most severe of cases, Alzheimer's and Schizophrenia may also be worsened in severity from an imbalance of this Chakra, as well as Bipolar disorder.

Mental/Behavioral Symptoms: A blocked Crown Chakra can lead to spiritual malaise. Isolation when you were previously a social butterfly one of the common symptoms of an issue with this Chakra. Joylessness, lack of inspiration, and even egomania can also occur with this blockage of this Chakra.

This is a basic list, however, you will learn more as you research on your own as well. As you can see, Chakra points indeed cover a wide range of bodily and mental functions. 'So, how do I use this information to mitigate a Chakra blockage?', you ask. There are a number of ways, not strictly relegated to meditation techniques, but related to the spheres of governance associated with each Chakra. Let's discuss what can be done to heal particular Chakras.

Healing a Chakra Blockage

1. **Root Chakra-** Healing a blockage with the Root Chakra can be accomplished in a number of ways. Examples of actions that you might take are as follows:

- As this Chakra is associated with home security as well as material goods, try to personalize your home a little once a week in a fashion that reflects you. Perhaps you have items that you collect that could be displayed in a more prominent place so that you may enjoy them more when you relax at home.
- As we have incorporated colors into our Chakra meditations, incorporate the color red into your house decoration or in your clothing scheme. The color association will keep the Chakra focus in your subconscious to help build its energy
- Use the meditation that we taught you previously, focusing on the Root Chakra. Tap the top of your head lightly every few

moments and visualize the color red as you do so. This association gives you a quick, mobile means of bringing up the energy of this Chakra when you need it, a mnemonic device that consists of simply tapping the top of your head a few times to invoke the memories and feelings of the meditation. This can be done with any of the Chakras.

- Cleaning your home is a simple means of feeding your Root Chakra. When your home is organized you will feel more comfortable and safe from the energy that you have provided to the Root Chakra.

2. **Sacral Chakra-** Blockage of the Chakra of emotional connections can be mitigated in the following ways:

- Volunteer work to bring yourself closer to others can help nourish your sense of closeness to the community. This, in turn, will strengthen your Sacral Chakra.
- Socialize! Invite some close friends for a night at your place. Have dinner with a friend once a week. Interface with others strengthens the Sacral Chakra. It may feel awkward at first but when you recognize that the problem is a Chakra imbalance and not the result of an outside influence then you will find it easier to spend time with others who are important in your life.

3. **Solar Plexus Chakra-** The Solar Plexus Chakra governs the sense of self, as such, blockages should be dealt with quickly. Here are some ways to accomplish this:

- Incorporate the color Yellow into your daily routine. Wear some gold or golden-colored jewelry if you have some. Yellow foods can empower this Chakra as well.

- Meditation with no specific aim but achieving a stillness of thought can promote self-contemplation, as you learn to listen rather than to always speak. This can empower the Solar Plexus Chakra as well.
- Begin keeping a journal. Committing our words to paper or other mediums helps to promote introspection of the self. At the same time, it gives you a record of feelings, moods, and general mindset at different points of time. This allows you to see the bigger picture when it comes to YOU. If you aren't the journal type, why not make more introspective posts in your Facebook? It's recommended if you do this that you turn off comments. This introspection is meant for you and should not be subject to comment or criticism, which could further block the Solar Plexus Chakra.

4. **Heart Chakra-** Influencing the ability to love yourself as well as our interpretations of life's lessons, blockage with this Chakra can cause a lot of chaos in your life. To remediate this, try doing one or more of the following to help re-energize and unblock this Chakra:

- Jewelry with green stones such as emerald, green tourmaline, or jade can help to energize this Chakra.
- Put some pictures of loved ones on display in your house, so that you have a daily reminder of those who are near and dear to you. Take a moment each morning to look upon them and recall a memory that makes up one of the thousands such memories that make you close.
- Blockage of this Chakra can interfere with your ability to give. Combat this in a simple way. Buy a friend a cup of coffee every now and again. Bring some donuts into the office for everyone. Donate to a local charity if you like. While it seems simple, the

act of giving is profound when it comes from the heart. Generosity is a sure way to strengthen this Chakra.
- Create a 'Book of Happy Memories'. Purchase a blank book at your local bookstore and leave it somewhere convenient at home. Try at least once a week to write down a happy memory in this book. Over time, they will add up, and you'll have a book that you can pick up and read at any time when it seems depression and the dark night are too much. This can chase away the shadows and the very act of writing these memories empowers the Heart Chakra greatly.

5. **Throat Chakra-** Ruling over communication with the self and others in speech, expression, and creativity, blockage of this Chakra is undesirable at the very least and can be crippling at it's very worst. To destroy a blockage of this Chakra, point the following exercises may be performed:

- If you find that you cannot speak so much, start making your words count. Speak only truthfully. Be blunt, honest, and succinct in all that you say. In this way, blockage of this Chakra can be mitigated at the same time that you are teaching yourself the immense power that economy of words can provide. Have you ever known someone in your life who spoke very little and yet every word was important, as if they'd carved their sentences with a razor to leave only what was meaningful? This exercise can help you to be that person and to revitalize the Throat Chakra
- Exercise your creativity. Writing, painting, sculpture, even making collages out of magazine cut-outs or extra photograph copies that you have can help to clear your mind. A portable means of this you will be familiar with from childhood... get a can of Play-Doh at your local department store. The non-toxic kids modeling clay is portable so you can keep it in your purse or

workbag and if you find your communication powers stymied from a Throat Chakra blockage, you can take it out and shape it to whatever you like. Whatever makes you smile. In this way you can capture some of the nostalgia of youth, when creative energies were at their finest and you had less cares from the weighty world trying to bring you down. These methods are an excellent way to strengthen your Throat Chakra.

6. **Third Eye Chakra-** Spiritual awareness, the ability to think logically and clearly, intuition... The Third Eye Chakra is as important to maintain in your life as any of the other 6 Chakras. Blockage can result in a number of ailments, as mentioned earlier in this chapter, but thankfully there are ways to deal with a blocked Third Eye Chakra. Try one or more of the following to restore energy to this important center of intuition:

- Visualization is one of the aspects of the mind that is affected by blockage of the Third Eye Chakra. An excellent but unconventional means of getting around this is to find yourself somewhere comfortable to sit so that you can exercise your imagination. What will we be visualizing? Try visualizing the absurd. It sounds odd, but this not only 'exercises' your visualization skills, but it can break the blockage to visualization that you are experiencing. Visualize a cat, sitting in a pie, holding the flag of your country. Visualize a bicycle racing down a hill with a large piece of cheese in the seat. Visualizing the unfamiliar and the absurd can strengthen your visualization skills and knock you out of the blockage that you are experiencing with this Chakra. Better, sharper visualization skills aid immensely in ensuring powerful meditation. So visualize the absurd, you'll be pleased with the results.

- Logic puzzles, such as Crossword puzzles or Sudoku contribute to structured, logical thinking. This is a fun and portable way that you can energize your Third Eye Chakra daily.
- Meditation in the woods, where you clear your mind of thought and absorb only the feel of the wind, the smells, and the sounds (without letting thoughts intrude, experience, do not narrate) can be an excellent way to achieve a feeling of spiritual awareness that requires no gods or churches. This also empowers the Third Eye Chakra.
- Keep an Intuition journal. Carry it in your purse, laptop, backpack, or whatever is convenient. When you get a feeling that you should do something, write it down and then simply listen to your intuition and do what feels right. Resist ignoring your inner voice for a week as an experiment. The important thing is to write down the results. Was your intuition correct? You'll find in most cases that indeed, it is.

7. **Crown Chakra-** The Crown Chakra exists as the seat of spiritual power. It controls the awareness of things around you on both the micro and the macro scale, which is to say it governs the details that you notice on coins in your collection, recognition of disruption in patterns on a design, or on a grander scale, the ability to see 5 or more moves ahead in chess or to eschew quick and expensive pleasures to save and build a business to sustain yourself in the long run. Thus, blockage to this Chakra can be devastating. The following methods can empower you to feed energy to your Crown Chakra to keep dissonance and blockage at bay. Give them a try and see for yourself.

- Weekly mindfulness exercise: Find yourself a comfortable seat by a window in your house or apartment that provides a scenic view or, barring that, go to a local park nearby where there will be many pleasant shapes, colors, sounds and scents to take it. Begin your breathing exercises to relax and start taking in your surroundings in a different, more unique way. Rather than assigning names to the things that you see, focus instead on their shapes and textures. Instead of seeing a dog and thinking 'Dog', try to view it as a collection of shapes. A tubular body, 4 rectangles, terminating at L-shapes for the feet. Is the fur matted or fluffy? What color is it? What about the trees? Some tall, some short, columns of brown with nerve-endings od green or, if it's autumn, orange, and red, and brown. Practice seeing things by the sum of their parts, broken down into shape, scents, colors, and sounds. When you see a person, instead of thinking 'That's joe', think 'Triangular nose, square head-shape, bow-legs... Avoid putting name to things and simply absorb their essence. Try doing this for 30 minutes or even 10, keeping the common-names out of your mind while focusing on the parts of life's clockwork that make them up. This powerful meditation can empower your Crown Chakra immensely. If you only do one exercise on this list, we recommend that you try this one. It's immensely powerful.

- Meditate on your Crown Chakra point in the same manner as the first meditation that we taught you. Simply discard the other Chakra focus and direct all of your attention to the Crown Chakra at the top of your head. See a white Lotus flower emerging at the center of the red light, growing bigger and bigger and more and more petals encircle it. The Crown Chakra is often symbolized as the Lotus with 1000 petals and so this meditation can strengthen your association with this Chakra at the same time that you are empowering it.
- Consider a Yoga class. Inverted Asanas are one pose that is associated with the Crown Chakra. Doing this pose daily before going to work in the morning can help to erode blockage of the Chakra and to strengthen it overall to prevent blockage in the first place.

So, now that we have a grounding in Chakra point history, Meanings, Meditations, and more, we'll focus the next chapter on assorted Chakra exercises that you can add to your growing knowledge of this powerful ancient science. After that, we're going to introduce you to Kundalini as a further means of self-empowerment. When you are ready, let's proceed.

Chapter 7 - Miscellaneous Chakra Exercises and More.

In this chapter we would like to provide you with more meditations and other tools to add to your Chakra toolbox. Experiment with the various exercises and meditations and feel free to customize them to you as you gain a deeper understanding of the Chakra system. In this way you will grow in health and spirituality more and more as you develop more knowledge of this most ancient science.

Let's begin with a means of carrying a bit of Chakra energy with you for when you need it.

Charging Chakra Stones

1. First we will need to collect a series of stones, either from nature (if you are lucky enough to have an assortment collected), your local gem and mineral shop, or EBay if you don't feel like leaving the house. Appropriate stones are as follows (This is, by no means, a complete list, so if you have or know of stones of the appropriate color, those will work just fine.) Get yourself one of each color and a small box or a bag to carry them in (which doesn't have to be fancy, anything from a leather pouch to a Crown Royal bag works just fine). Note, this exercise can also be done with jewelry if you have stones of the appropriate colors should you decide that you would like wearable Chakra stones.

- **Red** - Red Jasper, Ruby, and Bloodstone (This stone is red and green, so pick pieces that are largely red), Garnet, Rhodonite, and red Coral.
- **Orange**- orange Sunstone, Carnelian, orange Agate, orange Sapphire, Spessartine Garnet, Hessonite Garnet, orange Citrine, and Amber.
- **Yellow** - Yellow Citrine, Canary yellow Tourmaline, yellow (also called golden) Beryl, Gold, Iron Pyrite (Fool's Gold), Chrysoberyl, yellow Sapphire, and Lemon Quartz.
- **Green** - green Agate, Chalcedony, green Garnet, green Aventurine, Chrysoprase, Green Apatite, Emerald, Amazonite, Jade, Bloodstone, Hiddenite, Peridot, and Serpentine.
- **Blue** - Labradorite, Aquamarine, Blue Topaz, Blue Sapphire, Blue Lace Agate, Blue Apatite, Aragonize, Turquoise, blue Aventurine, Azurite, Benetoite, and Celestine.
- **Indigo** - Tanzanite, Indigo Crystal, Sodalite, Azurite, indigo Labradorite, and Iolite.
- **Violet** - Amethyst, violet Apatite, violet Sodalite. A large number of minerals may be found in violet as well, such as Spinel, Topaz, Beryl, Tourmaline, Barite, and Jadeite.

2. Now that you `have collected your 7 stones spend some moments studying each of them, memorizing what details stick out the most in your mind. Perhaps some have interesting, unique patterns, or particular brilliance in color. Pay attention to the textures as well. Are they smooth? Do you notice any chips or lines you can feel with your fingers? Once you have committed their look and feel to memory we can move to the next step.

3. Perform a variant of the first meditation which we have taught you. With each Chakra point, pick up the corresponding stone. Spend a few moments focusing on visualizing the energy from the

Chakra point. See the stone as well, seated at the center of power as if hovering in front of you or affixed to your skin. Say the Sanskrit name of the Chakra as you do this, repeating it in intervals as you visualize filling the stone with Chakra energy. The names again are as follows:

- Root Chakra - Muladhara
- Sacral Chakra - Svadhishthana
- Solar Plexus Chakra - Manipura
- Heart Chakra - Anahata
- Throat Chakra - Vishuddha
- Third Eye Chakra - Ajna
- Crown Chakra - Sahasrara

When you visualize the stone glowing with the same power that you see at the actual Chakra point, place it inside your box or bag and you may then proceed to the next stone.

4. Once you have energized all of the stones, aligning them with your Chakra energy, close the box or bag. You're done! When you feel you are blocked or imbalanced in a particular Chakra you now have a thing of beauty that you can carry with you to bolster your Chakra energies. Think of them as 'Chakra Batteries'. When you feel their efficacy is fading or they are 'losing their charge', simple set some time aside to repeat the exercise which you have just learned to re-energize them as-needed.

After the meditation that we've provided, we thought a bit of variety might be called for. As you adopt the lifestyle of Chakra power (and don't be fooled, when you've learned the efficacy of this system you will want to adopt it into your lifestyle) you will want to incorporate this wisdom into various aspects of your life. In the spirit of this, we've compiled a list of foods associated with the 7 Chakras so that you can strengthen your energies through their color associations at the same time that you are nourishing your body with delicious foods. Think of it as a culinary strategy for keeping in balance or strengthening a particular Chakra point.

Chakra Foods

1. **Root Chakra**- Color: Red

    - Strawberries, Cherries, Spaghetti with red tomato or meat sauce. Red Bell Peppers in your salad, tomatoes, red apples... Get creative. There are many red foods that will fill you up while you empower your Root Chakra.

2. **Sacral Chakra**- Color: Orange

    - Oranges, Tangerines, Cantaloupe... All good examples. If you fancy Chinese food, Sweet and Sour pork with orange sauce and Orange Chicken are also a delicious way to fill your stomach and prime your Sacral Chakra.

3. **Solar Plexus Chakra**- Color: Yellow

    - Bananas, Yellow Squash, and Corn are prime examples. Fresh pineapple and many types of yellow cheeses are also a healthy and smart way to empower your Solar Plexus Chakra by the medium of taste.

4. **Heart Chakra**- Color: Green

- Salad, Brocolli, Spinach, Green bell peppers, Green apples, Okra (and if you are from the Southern states of America, fried Green Okra is certainly close to your heart), and Honeydew are all good foods for powering this Chakra.

5. **Throat Chakra**- Color: Blue

    - A delicious bowl of Blueberries is a healthy treat that aligns with the color of the Throat Chakra.

6. **Third Eye Chakra**- Color: Indigo

    - Black Beans, and Plums are blue with black overtones, and thus they serve as a tasty meal or snack with a color receptive to your mind from your meditations on your Third Eye Chakra.

7. **Crown Chakra**- Color: Violet

    - Eggplant, Purple carrots, Concord grapes, Red Cabbage, and Purple Kale are all the correct hues for feeding the Crown Chakra while you feed yourself.

Now that you have the means to supplement your diet and you have created a portable set of Chakra stones. Let's discuss a mediation that you can do with crystals to align your Chakras. Crystals are a powerful means of aligning your Chakras. By their very nature, in the finer crystals you get a property known as a 'Crystal Lattice', which is a symmetrical three-dimensional alignment of atoms within and throughout the body of the crystal. As such, we may take advantage of this symmetry to bring about balance in our Chakras with the following exercise:

Crystal Chakra Alignment

1. First we need to obtain the crystals. Each item on the list below is an actual crystal containing the color properties coupled with the crystal lattice structure which is desirable for alignment of your Chakras. These may be obtained most easily through eBay or a local gem and mineral show.

- Root Chakra - Red - Rose Quartz
- Sacral Chakra - Orange - Orange Calcite crystal
- Solar Plexus Chakra - Yellow - yellow Citrine crystal
- Heart Chakra - Green - Dioptase crystal
- Throat Chakra - Blue - Celestine crystal (also known as Celestite)
- Third Eye Chakra - Indigo - Tanzanite crystal (look for the dark blue/black Indigo hues)
- Crown Chakra - Amethyst crystal

2. Once the crystals have been obtained, when you are ready to begin start by cleaning the crystals. Place them briefly in a solution of water and salt to purify them, followed by cleaning them under running cold water once the salt has done its purification job so that you are left with a residue-free, clean and purified crystal.

3. Find a comfortable spot at home or out in nature (take a sleeping bag to lay on top of if you don't have a soft surface, the backyard is fine if you don't have a private spot in the forest nearby).

4. Lay down on your back and begin your breathing exercises in order to put yourself in a relaxed and receptive state.

5. Begin placing the crystals on your Chakra points, reciting the Sanskrit name for each you place the crystal. The Crown Chakra crystal will go above your head but all of the others will be on your body. Do this slowly, visualizing the light at each Chakra

point blazing, lighting up the crystal which conducts the energy like the ancient circuit that it is. Envision the Chakra point in your body acquiring the symmetry of the crystal lattice, the energies aligning in your body.

6. Leave them in place and focus on visualizing all of the Chakras joining together into a mighty and complex symmetry. Traditionally it's viewed as a series of halo-like circles around the body, but let your imagination choose the form that it takes. Perhaps you see your Chakra energies as a large crystal encompassing you, with perfectly aligned crystalline layers inside, all of the appropriate colors. Go with your intuition and personal creativity.

7. Lay there for 5 to 10 minutes and then remove all of the crystals, placing them somewhere safe. We recommend obtaining a box specifically for them, as you will not be carrying them around and should only use these crystals specifically for this alignment exercise.

Now that we have explored a basic crystal exercise, another let's introduce another way that you can stimulate your Chakra points. Aromatherapy has been used for thousands of years as a means of promoting health and mental well-being. As it turns out, this has applications in stimulating the Chakras as well. Below is a list of essential oils which you may use to stimulate various Chakra points.

Chakra Essential Oils

1. **Root Chakra**

- Rosewood
- Frankincense
- Patchouli

2. Sacral Chakra

- Cardamom
- Jasmine
- Clary Sage

3. Solar Plexus Chakra

- Juniper
- Hyssop
- Pine

4. Heart Chakra

- Ylang Ylang
- Bergamot
- Rose

5. Throat Chakra

- Blue Chamomile
- Peppermint
- Lavender

6. Third Eye Chakra

- Lemon
- Rosemary
- Sandalwood

7. Crown Chakra

- Rosewood

- Frankincense
- Neroli

Alternately, bath salts of the same scents are a wonderful way to stimulate your Chakras as well while you relax and unwind. You can also anoint your Chakra stones with these oils to add a little extra charge or as an olfactory aid in your meditations on specific Chakras. Essential oils are an excellent addition to your growing collection of tools with which to enhance and unblock your Chakras, so consider acquiring them as soon as you can.

Now that we have gone into some Chakra basics to get you started we are going to move forward and discuss another powerful means of enhancing your life.

Kundalini. Don't know what that is? Don't worry. In the next chapter we will discuss what exactly Kundalini is, a little about its history, and what it can do for you. Let's move on to Chapter 8 get started.

Chapter 8 - Kundalini energy - Historical background and understanding Kundalini

So, we have learned about Chakra energies, now it's time to learn about another powerful energy that you can apply to your life many, many ways. We're talking, of course, about Kundalini. So what is Kundalini?

Kundalini is referred to often as 'The Serpent Power', because it's an energy that coils 3 and one half times at the base of your spine, terminating at the sacrum bone. Interestingly enough, The Egyptians and Greeks considered the Sacrum bone metaphysically significant. It's the last bone to burn during cremation and even the Latin name, 'Os Sacrum', suggests that it relates to the divine.

Your Kundalini energy coils at the base of your spine and nourishes the Tree of Life within all of us and can be used in conjunction with your Chakras or even on its own. It's considered a feminine energy. So, what can it be used for? We'll go a little into its applications in this chapter, followed by a chapter that will teach you how to prepare for a Kundalini awakening. Then we'll follow that up with exercises that you can utilize. First, however, let's go briefly into a little on the history and etymology of Kundalini.

Kundalini, like the Chakras, is first mentioned in the Upanishads. This means that it dates back to between 1000 and 1500 B.C..The Sanskrit root of the name, 'kundalin', literally translates as 'circular', reflecting the coil of energy from which the 'Serpent Power' description is formed. The energy is said to rise from the

Root Chakra when awakened, coiling around the spine to the top of the head. So, what is Kundalini awakening? Simply put, this is the time in your life when the Serpent energy becomes active. This can manifest in a number of ways and unfortunately, not all of them are pleasant. That said, recognizing a Kundalini awakening can help you to direct your attention to the development of this power in order utilize it in only beneficial ways.

Now, what are signs of Kundalini Awakening? There are a number of them which we will list. It should be noted, if you have experienced an awakening, you are very, very lucky. Less than half of the people in the world will experience one. Take advantage of this gift and develop this energy and your life will be all the richer and fuller for it. That said, here are some signs that you might be experiencing a Kundalini Awakening:

- A sudden awareness of destiny. You find that you know exactly what you wish to do with your life. What will be most fulfilling and conducive to happiness and personal growth. This can strike you out of the blue and is a powerful sign of a Kundalni awakening. That said, the inverse can also occur, as in our next example.
- Your life is suddenly falling apart. Everything that worked for you in your 'old' life, all the tricks and methods used to cope and succeed are suddenly failing you. This is not necessarily a bad thing, but it can be very trying. You will need to review various aspects of your life to decide what needs to be cut out. This is the start of your journey to the person that you are becoming. It will take courage and the support of friends but if you can keep your fears at bay and push forward then you will come out better for it.
- Anxiety and Insomnia from sudden bursts of energy can occur. Physical manifestations can include shaking. Doctors will likely

have no idea what to do or could prescribe you medications that you might not actually need. In such cases of a violent awakening of the Kundalini you will want to examine your Chakra and Kundalini energies through meditations so that you can learn to better conduct the flow of these sudden energies.
- Powerful intuition and spiritual understanding that you did not previously possess can occur. Usually it will manifest periodically in quick bursts, such as instinctively knowing that someone would be toxic or benevolent to you or you might experience occasional meditations that have more power than previously experienced. This is something that you will want to cultivate and we will tell you a number of ways that this can be accomplished in the following chapter.
- A sudden experience of divine bliss can occur. You suddenly understand, even if only for a brief moment, your place in the universe and everything. This is one of the more powerful signs of a Kundalini awakening.
- You may experience energy or an intense heat rising from the base of your spine to your Crown Chakra. This might occur during a particularly powerful meditation or even at a seemingly random time, like when you are out enjoying yourself in nature.
- Increased sensitivity may occur. You may find yourself noticing all the individual ingredients of the food that you are eating. You might suddenly find yourself in possession of sudden insight or a similarly advanced awareness regarding the behaviors of people in your life. You begin noticing the energies of particular places, both the good and the bad. This is another great sign of a Kundalini awakening and an indication that you should begin development of these energies right away.
- You find yourself suddenly obsessed with trying new things. Maybe you want to go skydiving all of the sudden or feel the

need to start going to the gym regularly. Maybe it manifests in a sudden urge to travel that you can't seem to shake. This is yet another powerful sign that your Serpent power has awakened.
- You become suddenly aware that it's your Ego that has been holding you back all of this time. This is good, as it gives you a chance to let go in order to become more at one with the life around you.

Now that we have described some symptoms that can indicate that you have had a Kundalini awakening, let's talk a little about the applications. Kundalini can be used to manipulate Chakra energy, for instance. Through the medium of Kundalini mantras, a number of things may be accomplished as well, such as protection from harm, increases in creativity, and the dispersion of fear and anxiety. Some other benefits of an awakened Kundalini that you might experience:

- Release of repressed thoughts and emotional 'baggage'.
- A heightened state of consciousness.
- You might find yourself aging more slowly, retaining a more youthful look than you would aging normally.
- An increased sense of perception can arise, where you are more sensitive to sights, sounds, smells, and colors.
- A strong sense of peace can enter your life.
- You may experience increased spiritual connections with the people and places around you.

These are just a few of the benefits that may occur with an Awakened Chakra. In our next chapter, we are going to discuss preparation for awakening your Kundalini so that you can be ready. As we've mentioned in this chapter, when the energy awakens it can be quite a powerful experience, so we want to make sure that you are fully prepared. It's very important that you do not skip these steps or you may experience some of the negative symptoms that we've previously discussed. Practice patience and you soon be able to experience your Kundalini awakening so that you can begin practicing the manipulation of this powerful energy. Let's proceed to the next chapter so that we may get you prepared.

Chapter 9 - Preparations and steps for Releasing your Serpent Power

If you have not already experienced a Kundalini awakening, there are way to prepare your body and mind in order to be both prepared and receptive to its release. In this chapter we are going to discuss these preparations so that you will be ready when the Serpent energy is awakened within you. First, let's go into preparations of the body.

Preparations for the Body

Preparations for the body are relatively simple. Here are 3 items that you should focus on to ensure that your body is prepared.

- Exercise for a week before proceeding so that your body is a healthier conduit for the energies.
- Try to avoid junk food, stick to salads and other healthier meals.
- Practice your breathing exercises. You will want to ensure that you can follow the proper breathing patterns without consciously having to count the moments when you inhale, hold, and exhale.

Preparations for the Mind

It's important that you prepare your mind for the awakening of your Kundalini energies. This is a bigger list of items, as it's very important to have your mind in order so that you can be receptive to the energies that will stir with your Kundalini awakening and to better avoid some of the pitfalls. There are the things that you will want to do:

- One week of daily meditation. There needs to be no focus to this meditation, only a clearing of the mind. Quiet all of your thoughts and simply let yourself listen, smell, hear, and feel the world around you. This will get you relaxed and in a proper mindset for proceeding.
- Be serious in your intent to awaken your Kundalini. This is not something that you can do halfway and its life-changing, so you need to be serious in your intent and firm in the knowledge that this is <u>exactly</u> what you want to do.
- Keep your mind free of emotional conflicts. Awakening of the Kundalini can be a jarring experience and if you are not capable of managing such feelings as anger, jealousy, or worry then you are not yet ready.
- Don't listen if someone ridicules you for wanting to do this. There are skeptics and other toxic personalities everywhere, minimize your contact with these people whenever possible. You know what is best for you.
- Balance your Chakra energy beforehand so that there is no blockage. Think of the Kundalini energy as a power generator. You wouldn't want to hook it up if some of the circuits were already fried, so be sure to perform the meditation for balancing your Chakras before you proceed.
- Understand that the energy may manifest destructively at first. Hopefully this will not be the case, but as mentioned previously in the list of symptoms of Kundalini awakening, sometimes anxiety or other undesirable 'side-effects' may result. Be ready to meditate or have your crystals at hand for Chakra alignment just in case you might need it. Above all, don't worry. There are a wide variety of reactions that one can have to the awakening of this energy and most likely it will be a positive reaction, still, be prepared.

Once you have prepared for a week with the steps that we have outlined, you should be ready for initiating the initial experience. If your Kundalini does not awaken the first time that you try, don't worry. You can always try again or, if needed, seek the help of a Guru to help you awaken this energy if it is proving truly resistant. If you do have to try again, wait a few weeks before you do. It's important not to try and force this energy awake. If it's unresponsive, there may be a mental or spiritual issue that needs to be dealt with before you can safely release this energy.

Now that we are prepared, let's proceed. We'll start with a necessary first step of Accessing your Central channel so that the energy will have somewhere to go (more about that shortly). We'll follow this with techniques that you may employ for awakening your Kundalini energy.

Accessing Sushumna Nadi (your Central Channel)

Your Central Channel is the Nadi, or 'energy channel' that is associated with your spiritual growth. It's important to empower this channel, as this is going to be used by your Kundalini energy. A means to activate this channel are as follows:

1. Go to your favorite comfortable meditation spot. Sit down, close your eyes, and begin your breathing exercises.

2. Focus on your Sacrum (at the base of your spine, close to the tailbone). Do this until you sense a thrumming or vibration of energy. Once you have have found it, begin repeating the following mantra. Sa Ta Na Ma. This mantra is called the Panj

Shabad (and we will go into mantras more in the next chapter, just so you know.). It translates out as 'Infinity, Life, Death, Rebirth' and is widely used by practitioners of Kundalini.

3. Feel the vibrating energy as it moves slowly up your spine. Visualize the energy filling your pelvic and abdominal areas. Let the energy push when it seems to reach its limit. See it increasing in capacity and size.

Now that you have prepared this spiritual center, we are ready to move on. to techniques

Techniques for Awakening your Kundalini energy

1. Begin your breathing exercises, but we are going to add a twist. You will want to visualize your breath as power, moving up from your Root Charka as you inhale, going next to the Sacral Chakra, Then to the Solar Plexus Chakra. Let it continue up to the Heart Chakra, the Throat Chakra, your Third Eye Chakra and finally, the Crown Chakra.

2. Hold the energy in place at your Crown Chakra for a few moments (depending on your chosen breathing pattern), and then when you exhale, repeat the process in reverse while chanting the Mantra 'Sat Nam'(One of the most widely used Mantras, this translates to 'Truth is my Identity'). Let the power pass from your Crown Chakra, to your Third Eye Chakra, then the Throat Chakra. Let it continue to the Heart Chakra, the Solar Plexus Chakra, the Sacral Chakra, and lastly, the Root Chakra.

3. As the Kundalini Awakening is generally performed by a Guru, we are going to do a little creative visualization in an attempt to negate this requirement. Visualize someone in your life or

someone that you have read about whom you consider a great spiritual teacher. This will align their energies with yours. Say their name as you inhale and exhale. If you are uncomfortable with this, you can say 'Enlighten me' instead. Feel the Serpent energy uncoiling as it moves up your body, empowering your Chakras and filling you with energy.

Should results not come for you with this particular method, now that you have accessed your Sushumna Nadi there are ways that you can attempt to coax an Awakening that are less-rushed. Here are some more techniques for you:

- If you are familiar with Kundalini Yoga, you can practice Asanas. Asanas are a great way to promote a Kundalini awakening (and useful for a number of other things as well.).
- Get some meditative music and dance to it. Let the music guide your dance. The mind state it produces it conducive to a Kundalini awakening.
- Daily Meditation can prepare one for the awakening of the Serpent power.
- Chanting Mantras can encourage a Kundalini awakening (and they are good for many different things, as we will discuss in the next chapter)
- Focus 1 hour a day on your hobbies or interests after performing the Sushumna meditation. This produces a focus on the self and can also lead to a slow and powerful Kundalini awakening.

Now that we have discussed preparations and techniques that may be employed for inducing a Kundalini awakening, let's move on to Chapter 10 'Kundalini Meditations and Exercises'. There we will discuss meditations and mantras that can help you to strengthen and grow your Kundalini energy, as well as discuss a number of different applications that you can employ in your life as well. Let's move on now and learn more.

Chapter 10 - Kundalini Meditations and Exercises

In this chapter we are going to teach you some meditations and Mantras that you can employ to exercise your Serpent power. There are a number of things that you can do with this energy and we will include examples of various forms of as we progress through this chapter.

So what are Mantras? How do I learn them and use them? First we are going to teach you a learning technique that will help you to learn Mantras (and anything else that you would like to learn, actually) quite quickly.

Learning Mantras

We're going to introduce you to an easy variation technique that makes learning quite simplified. This learning method is called 'Super learning' and it involves using music to open the left side of your brain, the side of creativity, while the right side, logic, learns as well. Things that you learn this way are not soon forgotten. You'll need a recorder (your laptop will work for this or you can use your cell phone).

Here are the steps:

- Record yourself speaking the Mantra or Mantras that you wish to learn. Speak with modulation of your voice. Sometimes say

the words high-pitched, other times with a bass rumble. It's important that the modulation of your voice patterns is many and varied. Don't speak in flat tones, rather, move your voice up and down in pitch and spectrum.
- Play some music, preferably instrumental, so that you don't inadvertently find yourself singing along.
- Sit comfortably and begin your breathing exercises.
- Listen to the recording while the music is playing. Repeat the words that you hear. The combination of the music and modulated voice patterns will help you to remember in a better, more powerful capacity.
- Once you know the Mantras by heart, you are ready to proceed to deeper meditations.

Now that you know how to learn them so that you can integrate Mantras into your meditations, here are some Mantras that you can use. There are more out there that you can search for, but consider this a primer, something to start with, until you are ready for more. Even the mastery of what we have provided here will add immense power to your life, indeed, you may need nothing more, but experience shows us that you will ever seek to learn more. As you should.

Without further ado, here are your beginning Mantras:

Mantras

We mentioned Mantras previously but haven't really gone into them in any detail. So, what is a Mantra? A Mantra is a 'sacred utterance', believed to have psychological or spiritual power. Typically, words in the sacred Indian language Gurmukhi, these words are said to have power, even when the meaning is not known by the one uttering them. We've compiled you a large list of Mantras, some that are in very widespread use by Kundalini practitioners and some that are a little more obscure. They serve a number of purposes, as you will see. Try adding Mantras to your meditations to direct focus and achieve desired effects.

1. **Mantra:** "Om"

Translation: No translation is given, "Om" is purported to be the first sound that was heard at the beginning of the existence of the universe.

Purpose: Arguably the most well-known word Mantra on this list, Om is a powerful sacred word that you can use during your meditations. As you say the word, see the Chakra points empowering themselves, starting from the Root and all the way up to the Crown. This Mantra is also said to increase your communications skills, as it unblocks and strengthens the Throat Chakra.

2. **Mantra:** "Akal, Maha Kal"

Translation: Undying, Great death.

Purpose: This powerful Mantra serves the purpose of removing fear and anxiety by relaxing the mind. Use it as-needed if you suffer from anxiety and you are sure to see improvements.

3. **Mantra:** 'Ong Namo, Guru Dev Namo'

Translation: 'I call upon the divine wisdom'

Purpose: Traditionally used before a session of Kundalini Yoga, this Mantra may also be employed before your standard meditation sessions as well. It's thought to attune the Practitioner's mind to wisdom.

4. **Mantra:** 'Ong Sohung'

Translation: 'I am the creative consciousness'

Purpose: This Mantra may be used to stimulate creativity and to open the Heart Chakra.

5. **Mantra:** 'Wahe Guru'

Translation: 'The ecstasy of undescribable, divine wisdom'

Purpose: This Mantra represents the ecstasy of divine wisdom. It may be used to increase one's organizational skills and for aiding in self-transformation. Use this Mantra in meditations early in your Kundalini practice to help develop your skills more quickly as you become more adept in Chakra and Kundalini energy manipulation. This Mantra also lifts the energy of the spirit.

6. **Mantra:** 'Sat Nam'

Translation: 'Truth is my identity'

Purpose: This is a powerful Mantra, sometimes described by the relationship between the seed and the tree. The seed is young and yet it contains all of the wisdom and majesty of the mighty tree that it's becoming. Invocation of this Mantra in meditation can assist you in focusing on your destiny as well as the awakening of your Kundalini energy.

7. **Mantra:** 'Har'

Translation: 'The Creative Infinity'

Purpose: This Mantra may be used in your meditations in order to inspire creativity. Focus on your Sacral Chakra to boost it with this

Mantra and you will have an overabundance of creativity to draw upon for your plans and projects.

8. **Mantra:** 'Hum Dum Har Har'

Translation: 'We are the Universe, the Creative Infinity'

Purpose: Promotes peace and tranquility, as well as stimulation of the Sacral, Third Eye, and Crown Chakras. Use this Mantra to stimulate them for targeted focus of these three Chakras and your Kundalini energy.

9. **Mantra:** ' Prana, Apana, Sushumna, Hari. Hari Har, Hari Har, Hari Har, Hari'

Translation: Prana is life-energy. Sushumna, as we mentioned before is the central channel, and Har is the Creative Infinity.

Purpose: This is a powerful Mantra for healing. In your meditations, as you chant the Mantra, feel healing energy flowing up from your spine and moving to afflicted areas which you wish to heal. These energies can assist you in healing more quickly, so be sure to learn and use this Mantra often.

10. **Mantra:** ' Ad Guray Nameh, Jugad Guray Nameh, Sat Guray Nameh, Siri Guru Devay Nameh'

Translation: 'I bow to the primal teacher who takes us to divine inspiration, I bow to the ancient wisdoms, I bow to the true and hidden wisdom.'

Purpose: This is a protective Mantra. When you feel that you are being polluted by toxic personalities or if you are suffering anxiety and to invoke wish spiritual protection, use this Mantra in a meditation. See a powerful white light surrounding you as you chant the words. This is another good Mantra to memorize.

11. **Mantra:** 'Gobinde, Mukunde, Udare, Apare, Haring, Karing, Nirname, Akame'

Translation: 'Sustainer, Liberator, Enlightener, Infinity, Destroyer, Creator, Without a name, Without Desire'

Purpose: This Mantra works with Heart Chakra meditations, helping you with empathy, patience, tolerance, and compassion. This is also said to balance disharmonies in the brain. Use this to achieve both compassion and focus as you empower your Heart Chakra with this powerful Kundalini Mantra.

12. **Mantra:** ' Sat Narayan, Wha He Guru, Hari Narayan, Sat Nam'

Translation: Hari Narayan is 'creative sustenance', as 'Narayan' represents the infinite shapes that water may acquire.

Purpose: This Kundalini Mantra may be evoked to promote healing and clarity of thought. If something traumatic or shocking has occurred and you are feeling imbalanced, then invoke this Mantra in meditation to center yourself and strengthen the health of your body.

13. **Mantra:** 'Ek ong kar sat nam siri wha hay guru'

Translation: Loosely, 'The Creator and Creation are one in the ecstasy and bliss of wisdom.'

Purpose: Known as the 'Adi Shakti', this Mantra is said to open one to the infinite consciousness of the universe. This Mantra can be used to energize the Solar Plexus and lessen the chains of ego, opening you more to the universe.

14. **Mantra:** 'Ra Ma Da Sa Sa Say Sohung'

Translation: Unknown

Purpose: This Mantra stimulates the healing factors of your body and mind through Kundalini energy.

15. **Mantra:** 'Sa Re Sa Sa'

Translation: unknown

Purpose: This Mantra is used for removing negativity through the power of the Creative Infinity.

16. **Mantra:** ' Har Har Har Har Gobinday'

Translation: Unknown

Purpose: This Mantra can be used to dispel negativity associated with over-contemplation of the past. Use this to surmount fears related to what was before so that you can push on to what will be.

17. **Mantra:** ' Dhan Dhan Ram Das Gur'

Translation: Unknown

Purpose: This Mantra invokes spiritual guidance through the energies of Guru Ram Das. Ram Das was

a powerful Sikh Guru of the 14th century (definitely worth a google). As mentioned in previous chapters, alignment with the energies of a powerful teacher can be beneficial. This Mantra in particular is used to invoke miracles in situations where no solution seems to be possible.

18. **Mantra:** ' Chattar Chakkar Varti'

Translation: Unknown

Purpose: This is a powerful Mantra for invoking courage. When anxiety or fears beset you, find a comfortable spot to sit down and meditate while chanting this Mantra. It will empower you to succeed through the banishment of your fears and worries.

19. **Mantra:** ' Ek Ong Kar'

Translation: 'The Creator and the Creation are one'

Purpose: This is a Mantra that may be used in coaxing a Kundalini awakening. It increases universal awareness and spiritual harmony. This Mantra is often weaved into other Mantras to increase these aspects of the Mantra' applications.

20. **Mantra:** ' Ardas Bhaee Amar Das Guru, Amar Das Guru, Ardas Bhaee, Ram Das Guru, Ram Das Guru, Ram Das Guru, Sachee Sahee.'

Translation: Unknown

Purpose: This is another Mantra invoking the enlightened energies of Guru Ram Das. It's used as a prayer mantra, used to combine the energies of the spirit, the body, and the mind in a combined focus for achieving the outcome for which you are praying.

Not all Mantras need to be in Gurmuhki, you can also use Mantras in English that you have made yourself or from quotes that you have found particular auspicious, inspiring, or found to contain other particular meanings to you. For instance:

1. **Mantra:** 'First I was three people. Who I was, Who I am, and who I was becoming. Now I am everything and nothing.'

Purpose: Use this Mantra to promote personal growth and oneness with the universe. As you chant the words, let your ego drain from you. Some ego is good, as it drives you, but an over-developed ego can hold you back. Be humble and willing to learn what the universe has to teach you.

2. **Mantra:** 'If I worry all night, then I will be tired in the morning when I must face this problem.'

Purpose: Based on an old Viking saying, 'If you spend all night worrying about the battle, then you will be tired in the morning when you must fight it.', this powerful affirmation can help you to drive out anxiety. Repeat the original or the variation that we have provided as you visualize the anxiety leaving your body during this meditation. This can help you to achieve the peace that you require to overcome the obstacles in your path.

3. **Mantra:** 'I desire to learn. I understand that I know nothing but I will teach myself to listen.'

Purpose: Chant this as you visualize each of the Chakras. Say their Sanskrit names as you perform the first meditation of the Chakras that we provided you. Keep all other thoughts from your mind. Instead on these, listen to the silence and let yourself learn on a more primal, fundamental level. The language of the spirit cannot always be put into words, sans the occasional poet that springs forth every now and then. Once you understand, it doesn't matter if you can put it into words or not. All that matters are results and a deep understanding of the Chakras and the self.

4. **Mantra:** 'Simplicity is key. The silence roars. The Wise will learn it's wisdom.'

Purpose: Tranquility and logic do not necessarily play well. That is one reason that we often envy the ignorant. They seem so happy. The reason is that, because of their natures, they do not over-think things. Learning to let go of your worries, your ego, and your focus can teach you how to recognize the variables that sit just on the edge of your perception. Embrace this. Stop your mind and your logic, for once. A bit of nostalgia is probably the best example of this mode of thinking. Remember the Roadrunner cartoons? Wile E Coyote would chase the Roadrunner everywhere, sometimes even following a false trail off of a high cliff. He would never fall until the Roadrunner pointed out that he was floating in the air, no longer on the earth. Let loose the lattice or rules and ordered thinking and your mind and spirit can float as well. It's absurd, yet profound, much like the rest of life. Try it for yourself and see the benefits of disassociation. Divine Bliss lies in being all... and nothing.

5. **Mantra:** 'The mighty oak towers above us all. Once, it was only an acorn, like me.'

Purpose: This Mantra reminds us that profound spiritual growth may be achieved by coaxing the tiny embers of a desire to be wiser and more spiritual. What was once simply burning coals sets the imagination and will aflame, transforming the dross of the self from materials into fuel, and further transforming the spirit into the wild energy it can be, like Fire. As you meditate upon this, see yourself transforming into the acorn (or a seed of your choosing if you have a plant that is sacred to you). Humble, you enter the darkness of the Earth. See the skies above you at the same time that you see the nourishing prison to which you have consigned yourself, in the knowledge and wisdom that you know it's what you need to grow. Contemplate this. For the seed, it's all darkness, wet, and fertilizer, until what was only the core of a life strives to the surface, breaks it, and rises to the sun. Let the Mantra remind you that those who are humble may grow powerful if they only understand that there is light beyond the inherent darkness that shapes us, exactly the way that we need to be shaped. After all, does not Nature teach us that birth is always painful? Use this meditation to increase your patience, endurance, and to achieve the peace that you need to use as sustenance as you grow like the mighty oak.

Chapter 11- The Third Eye: Understanding and Opening your Sixth Sense

We've included this chapter because this is an area of Chakra and Kundalini studies in which many are interested in. The Crown Chakra is the seat of spiritual energy, however, as we've discussed in previous chapters, the Third Eye is where spiritual awareness resides. Thus, empowerment of this Chakra can give one heightened intuition and a better understanding of the flow of the universe all around us. The Third Eye Chakra also heightens logic, as if it were a generous friend offering you something you want and a one mystery present. You know there is something good in the mystery box, you just have to learn to trust in your friend.

Opening the Third Eye can be complicated, however, so we have compiled together some information to help you prepare so that you will be receptive lo the stimulation of this Chakra and to its full awakening. Keep in mind that patience will be required on your part but with the proper preparation comes the proper results.

First, let's go into preparation. This is actually quite simple. There are a number of habits that you can incorporate into your life that will stimulate this Chakra and prepare you spiritually for it's awakening. Here are a few things that you can do to get started:

Preparation for Opening the Third Eye

1. **Get close to your Logic-** The Third Eye predominantly rules intuition, with logic as a second. This is not to say that the logic it imparts is fallible or weak. Quite the contrary, it sharpens like a laser. This is to provide contrast, not to dissuade you from following your intuitions. Realization of this is important when working with this Chakra. So absorb the logic, read your favorite philosophers of reason, watch your deduction CSI show if you fancy that. Absorb as much logic as you can so that you can appreciate the value of a honed intuition when you achieve it. Many people have triumphed in life and business by following their 'gut', so it's hard to argue the value of intuition. If you need an explanation that doesn't seem so metaphysical, consider this. Your mind processes information better than any computer that exists. It takes in all of the variables, while giving you only what you need. Is it not possible that intuition might be subconscious, high-level math, comprised of ALL of the variables that the brain has digested and considered in your moments of sleep and boredom? That this thing we call 'intuition' is a survival and growth variable that is there to serve you? It's worth a moment of contemplation.

2. **Practice your creativity-** Expression of your creativity feeds your soul and empowers the Third Eye and the Throat Chakras. If you like to write, paint, or otherwise create in some form or fashion, then exercise this. One particular exercise helps you to practice intuition while expressing yourself artistically. Go to a secondhand bookstore and dredge up a collection of magazines. Get some poster board at your local grocery store and some glue. Try taking pictures of individuals and cut out pictures that you associate with them and paste them around the individuals picture. Pick someone you don't know a lot about already, so that

later when you have finished your collage you can read a quick biography on them through the magic of Google. See is the items that you associated with them are actually associated in real life. Don't worry if you only get a few things right at first. This is an exercise to flex spiritual muscles that you haven't been using. Sometimes this exercise can pleasantly surprise you.

3. **Meditate daily whenever possible-** Meditation is a good way to get in touch with the spiritual at the same time that you are helping yourself to relax and become at one with the universe around you. Focus specifically on the Third Eye Chakra, seeing an opening light in the space on your brow between your physical eyes. Visualize the world that is around you behind your closed eyes and see if any particular portions draw your attention. Open your eyes briefly and see where your attention has been drawn. Note the environment and contemplate what you have just seen with your eyes once again closed. As the Third Eye Chakra also associates with wisdom it's quite possible that you will find yourself gathering a deeper perspective of your environment while exercising your Third Eye Chakra in this manner. Give it a try and see for yourself.

4. **Detoxify your Pineal Gland-** Located at a level with your eyes in the center of the brain is your Pineal Gland. Yogis have studied and explored the connections with this gland and your Third Eye Chakra. Often viewed as the seat of the soul, taking steps to ensure the health of your Pineal Gland can, in turn, empower your Third Eye Chakra. There are certain steps that you can take to cleanse and detoxify this gland. They are as follows:

- Apple cider vinegar. Get the kind in a glass bottle. A spoonful a day can help to cleanse and refresh the Pineal Gland.

- Iodine - Seaweed, kelp, and various algae are a natural source of Iodine that can be used for detoxifying your Pineal Glands. They work by causing the excretion of heavy metals from the body. If you aren't a big fan of Sushi, you can purchase supplements that you can take via a dropper to get the Iodine that you are needing.
- Shilajit - Hailing from the Himalayan mountains, this is plant material that was preserves over millions of years. Containing more than 85 different trace minerals, this particular compound not only helps your Pineal Gland but is said to have Anti-Aging benefits as well. Search for it on Google, this might just be the supplement for you.
- Fulvic acid - The American version of Shilajit, 5 or 6 drops of this in water will let this plant-based supplement provide detoxification and daily maintenance of your Pineal Gland.
- Turmeric - This supplement can assist the Pineal Gland by helping to reduce the damage from fluoride exposure. Easy to obtain, this is definitely an item to add for detoxifying your Pineal Gland.
- Chaga Mushrooms - Widely hailed and used by the Japanese, Chinese, and Russian peoples, this mushroom has a number of qualities that are useful and beneficial. A natural producer of Melanin (which the Pineal Gland uses to help shield us from UV light), this mushroom is also considered an anti-tumor agent, as well as a booster of the immune system and good for the health of the central nervous system as well. Traditionally ingested as a tea, do a Google search on this yourself to see more of the benefits that come with this potent little mushroom. A number of scientific studies that been done on this one so you are in for a good read and some good health in your future.

Now that you've done some basic preparations, how does one actually go about opening the Third Eye? Not so fast, friend. First we need to consider the dangers of opening the Third Eye.

Primarily, there is a worry when opening the Third Eye of falling prey to delusion. You will have an influx of new data coming to your mind that you need to interpret. To avoid this, take everything very slowly. Intuition is a metaphysical muscle that needs to be flexed and grown, so don't start buying scratch-off cards or worrying over your flights until you've had time to develop your growing intuition. This is the process of a lifetime, so be patient. You'll reap immense benefits in Business and your Personal life but don't expect results 'overnight' and be careful about your early intuitions. Think of it in a work perspective. Sometimes you work with charts or graphs that contain an abundance of information. Were you able to understand them immediately or was there a learning curve?

Give it time and remember that every massive Oak tree you've ever seen started as a tiny acorn you could have crushed with your shoe.

Now that we've discussed the safety factor, what are the benefits of a well-developed Third Eye? They are as follows:

- Increased perception.
- understanding of your destiny.
- the ability to see the direction of your life as if reading it in a biography, constantly writing itself.
- Increased 'Luck' from your inner knowledge of the hidden variables around you.

At this point, we should be ready to go into techniques for opening the Third Eye, but first, in case of emergency:

Closing your Third Eye

1. Find a comfortable place to meditate.

2. Begin your breathing exercises.

3. Begin meditation. Visualize your Third eye. Flood it with visions of logic and art, such as mathematics, books, painting, and sculpting. The goal of this exercise is to route our intuition into logic and creativity if we are receiving headaches, strange dreams, or other effects from the awakening intuition. Logic especially is an important part of your Third Eye. You are actually exercising that Chakra every time that you use Google or read up on a subject that you are interested in. That said, drowning out intuition with a flood of facts can help you to push your Third Eye into a 'dormant' state. See the facts closing in, visualize the right side of your brain, the side associated with logic, flashing in bursts of light. Then say 'Let Intuition come later.' and visualize the Intuition energy as an Indigo glow, flowing into your left side of the brain. Complete the meditation by stating, 'Let my Intuition manifest as Creativity until I am ready for more.'. See the rest of the energy flowing into the left side (creativity associated) of your brain and see the glowing eye between your brows closing.

4. Now you have closed the Third Eye. Be careful, do this no more than once a month, you must let some intuition flow until you are ready again to accept the additional information. Intentional blockage for long periods of time of the Third Eye can lead to headaches and worse, so if you have to close it, then do so, but do it with the understanding that you must master this Chakra and learn to interpret the data that it sends to you.

We have discussed dangers, benefits, and methods of protecting yourself in an emergency, so we feel that you are finally prepared for opening your Third Eye to see what it can offer you. Here is a solid method for this that you can practice at home:

A Technique for Opening the Third Eye

1. Find a comfortable spot for meditation. This will take 30 minutes to an hour, so make sure that it's a good one.

2. Begin with your breathing exercises to get relaxed.

3. Perform the Crystal purification of your Chakras.

4. Meditate upon strengthening each Chakra, from Root to Crown to bring yourself a balance after the purification.

5. Following this, focus on your Third Eye Chakra. See the 'eye' shape between your eyes opening, showering the world around you in a discerning light. You will notice that everything that you perceive is sharper all of the sudden. Don't be afraid, go with it. Let the details come.

6. In lieu of a Manta, speak the following words, 'I do not understand all that I see, but I notice everything. I seek the wisdom to understand what I do not comprehend now.'

7. See your Third Eye light like a spotlight, circling around you, bringing in details that you missed before.

8. Close the meditation with a statement, 'Forever vigilant, I see and strive to understand. I will trust what I learn.'

Congratulations. You have opened your Third Eye Chakra. At first the information will seem to be too much. Don't let that worry you. Compare it to the color spectrum. If you were describing the scale of the colors of the Rainbow to a blind man or woman, how would you describe Indigo? 'A light and dark blue and black hue, not quite blue or purple? ' Explanations are hard to get concise, at first, but if you keep exercising your creativity and learning what the Third Eye has to teach you, then you will ascend from pupil to teacher in time. The woods are daunting if you are not a creature of nature, so let the information flow to you from your Third Eye and use it, trust it. Don't deceive yourself but take good opportunities. You will soon know the difference.

Now that we have discussed the pitfalls and pluses of empowering the Third Eye, let's move on to crystal and other healing techniques in the realms of Chakra and Kundalini.

Chapter 12 - Energy Healing with Crystals and Other Stones

One system used with both Chakra and Kundalini (as well as many other practices) is the healing power of various stones and crystals. We discussed in a previous chapter how to create Chakra stones, to energize and unblock your Chakra, points, as well as crystals for cleansing them. Now we would like to go into the healing properties of various stones so that you can acquaint yourself with them and add them to your meditations for greater efficacy and results. To this effect, we have compiled a list for you that includes the healing and other properties of crystals and various stones as well. They are as follows:

1. **Agate-** This stone is a powerful enhancer of cognition. Helping to produce clarity of thought, this is a good one to have nearby if you suffer from anxiety, wish to excel in social conversation, or wish to remediate other conditions that result in disorganized thought patterns.

2. **Amazonite-** This stone is particularly beneficial. It can be used to balance and cleanse all of the Chakras, as well as providing the healing benefits of keeping infection at bay as well as helping to clear up skin conditions.

3. **Aventurine-** Increasing recovery time, this stone is also good for the heart and the blood. As it's associated with the Heart Chakra, this can also be used to stimulate this energy center as well as to increase compassion and empathy.

4. **Amethyst-** Associated with the upper 3 Chakras (Throat, Third Eye, and Crown), this stone is good for healing conditions governed with this area. Headaches, neck pain, insomnia, and more. Get a nice Amethyst geode to put next to your work computer. Your workmates will admire the beauty without wondering the purpose (a nice geode is a fantastic thing of beauty) while you reap the health benefits.

5. **Bloodstone-** This reddish-green form of chalcedony promotes good circulation, as well as invigorating the revitalizing the body. If you exercise regularly, this can aid in your endurance to help you to sculpt and shape the body that you desire. Interestingly enough, this stone is said to have protection qualities as well. If your child is getting bullied at school, you can have them carry it or make a necklace to help calm those around them and to boost the child's system (in cases of fight or flight).

6. **Blue Topaz-** This stone has powerful properties that you can take advantage of. It's beneficial to mental illness, as well as issues of taste and sight. Use this for lessening of the vision, the palate, or distracted cognition. Easy to hide, this is a popular stone for jewelry, so you can keep it close without question.

7. **Citrine-** This stone may be used for issues of digestion, as well as stimulating your metabolism and strengthening nerves so that messages from your brain fire with an empowered rapidity. This is another jewelry stone, easy to hide, and easy to incorporate into your life.

8. **Fluorite-** Good for allergies, sinus infections, and mental acuity/focus, this is another good stone to add to your collection. Fluorite can alleviate inflammation and give you that extra focus edge that you need when focusing. Keep it close to you during

meditation in order to maximize the retention of the deep understandings and revelations that occur. There is nothing worse than forgetting something profound, hard-won, so consider Fluorite in the form of a necklace or even just in your pocket to retain those memories and to sharpen your focus.

9. **Hematite-** This stone helps you to resist anxiety. It promotes heart health, circulation, and is also associated with the organs of the root Chakra. You can also use it to relieve stress in sexual matters. Add this stone to your collection and you can see it's efficacy for yourself. You will not be disappointed.

10. **Jade-** This stone is associated with the Heart Chakra. It can aid in recovery after surgery, as well as act in a capacity of healing toxins of the blood. This stone aids in increasing compassion, empathy, and easing joint pain as well. Pretty stone, powerful influence. This is a good stone to keep close.

11. **Obsidian-** This is more a stone for mental than physical healing. Obsidian knives came before bronze and iron in many cultures. Still surgically sharp, some obsidian knives are sharper and more resilient than modern scalpels. A genuine icon of the past, Obsidian helps you heal the woes of the past. Get one. Look into its black sharpness, polish it, make a blade if you like. Let it remind you that the past cuts the sharpest but it's, indeed, only the past. This is a good one to make a necklace of. Its lesson needs no explanation. It cuts always and stays in the shadows. Let the dark do what it's supposed to, let it hide things and put them where they belong, because you won't walk far along a path if you walk looking behind you all of the time.

12. **Opal-** Opals are so fragile. They often provide floating images, tricks of the eye and mind. Illusions. As such, they are the perfect

stone for issues of the eye. Dimness of vision, loss of detail sight, these are things that can benefit from the procurement of a good opal. It doesn't have to be gemstone quality... indeed, poor quality Opals, even raw, have an aesthetic that reinforces the belief in what they can do. Look into raw or basic opals.

13. **Quartz-** One of the most common stones that also contains an abundance of power, Quartz may be used to boost the immune system, as well as the rest of the body. Clear, symmetrical... It's a perfect example of a refined crystal lattice. If you live in the USA, do a Google on crystal mines in Arkansas. For 10 to 15$, you can pick up crystals by hand brought fresh from the mines daily. Wear gloves, because raw crystal cuts like glass, but a little trip to Arkansas can get you hundreds of dollars worth of crystals for 10-15 per hour of your time with discerning eyes, gloves, and a bucket.

14. **Rose Quartz-** Associated with the Root and Heart Chakra, this crystal has many beneficial properties. Blood pressure, Tachycardia, this a useful stone to incorporate into your collection.

15. **Ruby-** Stimulating the Root Chakra, the Ruby is also a powerful stone for healing. It can help with issues of the heart as well as sexual dysfunction. It can increase focus and concentration and also promotes love.

16. **Sapphire-** Sapphire stimulates the Throat and the Third Eye Chakras. It can be used to prevent fever and is also good for ailments of the eyes. Its spiritual properties make it a good stone for the cleansing of the Chakras as well. As it is a jewelry stone and associated with the upper Third Chakras, this is a good stone

for earrings if you would like to wear them close to the Chakras that Sapphire affects.

17. **Shungite-** This rare stone is said to reduce the effects of EMF (electromagnetic frequency). You can place it close to electronics, such as cell phones and laptops, or other items that you use daily in order to reduce the EMF effects. Shungite also has detoxifying qualities. It can speed up detoxification and help to soothe the anxiety that comes so often with this process.

18. **Tanzanite-** Another jewelry stone, Tanzanite promotes psychic ability. It also is a powerful healing stone, promoting regeneration of skin, cells, and hair. It provides clarity and calm for meditation but is also said to help the comatose in finding their way home. Tanzanite is also said to be good for alcoholism and for lessening the pain from migraine headaches. A powerful stone, indeed.

19. **Tourmaline-** Strengthening the spine, the immune system, your adrenal glands, and your heart, this stone can also assist with easing stress and helping you to remove tension from your life.

20. **Turquoise-** Turquoise is associated with your Throat Chakra and can help with issues associated with the throat, ears, the neck, and even the brain. It's also good for achieving deeper meditations and stimulates the intuition, so this is a good stone to carry with you at all times.

If this seems like a lot of information to process, don't worry. A great way to learn the properties of your stones and to store them easily is this. Get yourself a fishing tackle box. It sounds a little unorthodox but give us a moment to explain. A tackle box contains a number of compartments, staked over one another, that you can pull out to take advantage of the modular storage capabilities. Get some note cards and scissors and cut out some squares of card that you can put at the bottom of the containers. Write the name of the stone and key words that tell you their properties. For instance, you might write 'Bloodstone -Endurance, Circulation, Exercise'. Later you can always adopt a jewelry box (or simply use it for the fancy ones) but a tackle box is actually quite good in that it can keep your stones separated, in good condition, and keep them from scratching each other as they would if they were simply all together in a box. If you prefer a more aesthetic approach and have a little talent in making new things, line the compartments with velvet, glue some brass or other items to the lid, and transform the box. Or you can spend a little extra time to make a wooden one with the same qualities (and some jewelry boxes already have the same type of storage). In the meantime, to save money and accomplish the same effect, get yourself a tackle box. They are also less likely to be stolen.

So, how do I use these stones?

Simply carry them with you or integrate them into jewelry. 'I can't make jewelry and it's expensive to have it made'., you say. Do yourself a favor and thank us later with this little trick. Go to Google and look up 'jewelry settings'. There are a number of talismans and other, more basic settings, just waiting for you to provide the stone. For instance, Google 'Garnet cabochon' and you will find round Garnets with a flat base, a sphere cut in half. You can easily put one of these in a setting by simply placing it and maneuvering the tongs in place by pushing them with pliers or in some cases, simply superglue it in place. Artistic expression strengthens the Throat and Third Eye Chakras, so why not give it a try?

You might find that you had a talent that you didn't know about.

If I use more than one stone will the energies conflict?

No. These stones are not people. They are energies of nature. Created over spans of time older than our civilizations, they are pure and produce only good and beneficial energies. Think of them like money. In Viking runes, money is simply mobile power that must be put into place and circulated. different stones are different currencies but their value does not diminish when you pile them together. They all convert into the power that you need and their difference is simply in their aesthetics. The only worry is that you may get too much of the energies that you are attempting to cultivate, so mix and match wisely. You will learn with experience.

Do I need to prepare them in a special way?

Stones, crystals, and minerals predate you enormously. They don't need a lot of care. If you wish to energize them, the way you would energize your own body for exercise, consider the following:

- Sunlight can energize your crystals, stones, and minerals.
- Moonlight works as well.
- Salt water clears out negativity.

- The smoke from smudge-sticks, lavender and sage, for instance, can purify your stones if you feel that they are losing their efficacy.

Some stones, such as Kyanite, need no purification. So do a little creative Googling. If you made a tackle box, a red stripe in the corner of the description can show you at a glance which stones should be purified weekly for best results.

Chapter 13 - Chakra Meditation Garden

We've spoken about the benefits of foods in cultivating a proper mindset. Foods of certain color have a psychological association with your understanding of the Chakra points. One way that you can nourish your mind and your energy centers is to create a garden. A small square of place in the backyard where you encourage and watch as foods and flowers of the appropriate colors grow.

This is a means to encourage your patience and to show you that your efforts, however big or small, bear merits while providing a peaceful place to meditate. This is how you will accomplish such a thing:

Prepare for yourself a garden. The following items are the colors that you will need:

Red foods: Tomatoes, Strawberries, Red peppers, Raspberry, Radish

Red Flowers:

- Red Cardinal- Blooming from Summer to Fall, these flowers have a lovely trumpet shape to them that is pleasing to the eye. These flowers also attract Hummingbirds.
- Red Roses- Longtime symbol of love, the tending and caring of a rosebush is relaxing and good for the soul. Consider planting a rosebush, it can bring you much enjoyment in future years.
- Red Petunia- Petunias are interesting flowers. While their red hues can indicate love or passion, depending on the setting they can also be used to represent anger or distaste with

something that a person has done. That said, their beautiful hues can add a nice bit of color to your garden, so consider Petunias.
- Red Pygmy Water Lily- Flowering from June to September, this beautiful lily is native to Meghalaya. Perfect for a koi pond or just a regular pond.
- Red Lilies- Like Roses, Red Lilies are also a powerful symbol of passion and love. They are a beautiful addition to any garden as well, so consider them for your meditation garden.

Orange foods: Oranges, Pumpkin, Carrot,

Orange Flowers:

- Begonias-Blooming in many colors, Begonias are a nice addition to any garden and easy to take care of.
- Marigolds- Blooming all summer long, Marigolds require a lot of sunlight but they can bloom in just about any soil, so if you need something pretty that grows in hardy climes, consider the Marigold.
- Tulips- Tulips are a good addition to your Meditation garden. You can also find them in virtually every color of the rainbow, so Tulips are a good choice if you are looking for a single type of plant to care for.
- Gerbera Daisies- These flowers come in many colors, including the Orange that represents the Sacral Chakra point. A nice addition to your garden.
- Daylilies- Despite their fragile appearance, these flowers grow and spread quickly. Thriving in partial shade or full sunlight, these are a wonderful addition to your meditation garden.

Yellow foods: Corn, Squash, yellow Bell Peppers

Yellow Flowers:

- Sunflowers - Hardy, easy to take care of, and lovely to look at, Sunflowers are a great addition to your garden and easy to take of as well.
- Water Lilies - Representing fertility and rebirth, these are a great addition to any garden pond.
- Dahlia- Popular in Victorian times, the Dahlia represents strength and elegance and is quite lovely to look at. A great addition to your Meditation garden.
- Lotus- One of the more delicate flowers, a Lotus is a powerful symbol of spiritual enlightenment and looks elegant in a backyard pond.
- Yarrow- Representative of love and healing, Yarrow is easy to cultivate and looks great in your garden.

Green foods: Green beans, Green Onions, Green Apple, Broccoli, Spinach

Green Flowers:

- Hydrangeas- Available in blue, pink, red, and green Hydrangeas are lovely and easy to care for. Consider them when planting your garden, you'll be happy that you did.
- Bells of Ireland- Easy to obtain and hardy, Bells of Ireland actually originated from Turkey. Easy to take care of and noted for their longevity, these are a great addition to any garden.
- Zinnia- Available in many colors, Green Zinnias are lovely to look at both inside and out of the home.
- Dianthus- This makes great borders for your garden. Dianthus is easy to raise and another of the hardy plants from this list.
- Mint- Great for teas, Mint adds color and scent to your Meditation Garden, enhancing the overall peacefulness.

Blue foods: Blueberries

Blue Flowers:

- Blue Hydrangeas-Hydrangeas have an amazing assortment of shadings, depending on the alkalinity of the soil they are growing in. Powder blue, sky blue, and deeper shades as well. Add them to your garden and enjoy.
- Blue Dandelions- Native to Asia and Europe, Blue Dandelions are becoming popular in the U.S. as well. Representative of happiness and tranquility, they are a fine addition to your meditation garden.
- Grape Hyacinth- Associated with rebirth, this plant grows in pleasant clusters and has a notable bulb shape quite unlike any other.
- Crystal Fountain Clematis- Associated with faithfulness, this climbing plant is an excellent addition to for providing a fine, dark blue hue to your garden.
- Bellflowers- Also known as 'Fairy Thimbles', these bell-shaped flowers are a lovely shade of blue that you can use to stimulate your Throat Chakra.

Indigo foods: Eggplant, Purple carrots.

Indigo Flowers:

- Indigo Tinctoria- Also known as 'True Indigo', this plant is a member of the bean family and is the source of the original Indigo color dyes.
- Blue False Indigo- Once used by Native Americans in making blue and indigo dyes, the blooms of this plant are stunning and a worthy addition to any garden.
- Mountain Larkspur- Larkspur is beautiful, but poisonous, so handle with care if you choose to add this to your garden.

Violet foods: Sweet purple onions, Purple Cabbage

Violet Flowers:

- Violet- It doesn't get more violet than violets. Add them to your garden to stimulate the Crown Chakra while you relax and mediate.
- Catmint- Requiring very little care, Catmint is lovely easy to raise.
- Verbena- Occurring in shades of magenta and violet, these bloom in summer and will last throughout it if roper care is taken of them.
- Canterbury Bells- Easy to raise and a joy to look upon, these come in many colors and have an attractive, bell-like shape.
- Sea Thistle- Often found wild in parts of the U.S., this plant is good for attracting butterflies and birds to your garden.

These are just a small sampling of flowers that you can cultivate in your garden. For best results, local plants are easier to obtain and already suited for your environment. That said, if you have a bit of a green thumb, the extra effort is really worth it. Cultivating a place for your meditations is definitely worth the time.

Chapter 14 - Kundalini and other Yoga forms

We wanted to include a chapter on another means of raising your Kundalini energy. Kundalini Yoga is quite excellent for this and a great way to keep in shape. So, what do we need to now to get started?

First, a little bit of history. While it's exact origins are unknown, earliest mentioned are attributed to the Upanishads. Traditionally taught from teacher to student, Kundalini yoga was not 'officially' adopted in the west until the late 1960's, when it was introduced commercially by Harbhajan Singh Khalsa, also known more popularly as Yogi Bhajan. Taking advantage of the 60's and 70's counterculture environment, Yogi Bhajan was in a good place to spread his message and his brand of Yoga spread as across the U.S. and Canada after he established a teacher training program in 1969.

As these teachings were normally passed on by word of mouth, from teacher to student, there was always some contention as to whose form of Yoga is the most 'pure.' Critics such as Virsa Singh, who practices the Gobind Sadan path of enlightenment have cited that in its earliest stages of developments, Yogi Bhajans form of Kundalini Yoga appears to be a mixture of Sikh Mantras, Tantric references, and Yogic postures. Gobind Sadan is a form of Sikhism that embraces, among other things, respect for all religions due to that person's particular belief in those systems. So, who is right?

The right system for you is the one that calls to you. For now, it's better to just focus on getting started. Kundalini yoga has attracted a growing number of practitioners for its health and spiritual benefits. We would humbly suggest that the best path is going to be steeped in traditions and yet unique for you, just as every spirit is unique.

So what's it all about?

Yoga consists of adopting various poses of the body in order to stimulate specific energies and/or to promote peace, self-awareness, and good health.

Other types of Yoga that you may have heard of include:

1. Ashtanga Yoga

Origin and Philosophies: The name, 'Ashtanga', comes from the Sanskrit word 'Asanga' mentioned in the Yoga Sutras of Patanjali. Meaning 'Eight Limbed', it referred to the Eightfold path of Yoga. Strict in its postures, this Yoga combined associated breaths with every stance in order to link the breath with every movement. While recorded in early manuscripts, this form of Yoga was introduced to the West in 1948 by K. Pattahbi Jois. Considered it a modern day version of traditional Indian teachings.

2. Hatha Yoga

Origin and Philosophies: Developed originally by a 15h century Hindu Sage named Yogi Swatmarama, the word 'Hatha' derives from 'Force'. Just about every Yoga pose taught and practice in the United States derives from Hatha Yoga and, as such, it's often used more as a generic term in the West for any type of Yoga involving physical poses. This Yoga chiefly employs asanas, which are Yogic poses, in order to better link the body and the mind as one.

3. Jivamukti Yoga

Origin and Philosophies: Jivamukti Yoga is a relative newcomer in this group, first developed in the by David Life and Sharon Gannon in1984 and comes not only with own poses but with spiritual and ethical tenets as well. The 5 tenets of Jivamukti include:

- Ahimsa- A Nonviolent lifestyle imparting kindness to animals, extending to vegetarianism, veganism, and animal rights.
- Bhakti - Self-Realization is accepted as the goal of Yoga.
- Dayana- Observation of Meditations
- Nada- Deep listening with music or even guided meditations.
- Shastra- Study of the ancient Yogic teachings

4. Iyengar Yoga

Origin and Philosophies: Created in 1966 by B.K.S. Iyengar, working in turn with by K. Pattahbi Jois, the creator of Ashtanga Yoga, Iyengar was first detailed in a book called 'Yoga Light'. This book quickly became a bestseller, as it focuses on a light form of Hatha Yoga, incorporating over 200 traditional poses, yet also incorporates the use of slings, blankets, belts and more in order to minimize risk of injury at the same time making the system accessible to Practitioners of any age or physical shape. This Yoga is strongly based as well in the eight-limb Yoga traditions of Patanjali in his test, 'Yoga Sutras'

5. Bikram Yoga

Origin and Philosophies: First developed in 1973 by Bikhram Choudhury, this Yoga is the most rigorous of the list. Focusing primarily on utilizing the Hatha techniques for exercise (sometimes in heated rooms), this Yoga is more about getting a physical workout.

So what about Kundalini Yoga?

Kundalini Yoga is a very different experience from the others. As we proceed further into this chapter we'll discuss a number of poses and exercises that you can do in order to take advantage of this wisdom for yourself. These are a few traditional exercises learned and taught by Yogi Bhajan and used daily around the world. Due to the enormous amount of material available on this subject we are only including a few poses and tips, just enough to get you started, in the interest of covering more subjects that we feel might be of interest to you in this book.

For our first exercise, we'll introduce you to the 'Frog' position.

Frog's position: 'To do the Frogs position, Squat down on your toes, heels touching, and your hand between your legs in front of you. Just like a frog sits. Raising your buttocks, slowly rise up, moving your head down towards your knees. They take a little practice, but Frogs are a great way to stimulate the Root and Sacral Chakras. Do 26-52 Frogs in the morning and you'll feel the difference.

Crow Squats: Next we will try Crow Squats. Like Frogs, Crow Squats stimulate the First and Second Chakras while also improving your circulation. Squat down, with your hands held straight out in front you or fingers-locked together on the top of your head. Slowly come into a standing position and repeat 26-52 times.

Triangle pose: This pose stimulates the Pituary gland and also good for your spine. Stand with your feet apart at about a hip-width. Bend over, placing your arms about 3 feet in front of your feet. Raise your buttocks so that you are adopting a triangular shape in this pose. Hold this position for 3 to 5 minutes, breathing deeply so that you stay relaxed and in proper form.

Chakras Ana: This pose energizes all of your Chakras. It's a little tricky to do. Laying on your back you will want to place your hands on the sides of your head, fingers pointing towards your toes. Slowly raise, so that your body makes the shape of an arch. Hold this pose for 30 seconds and then slowly lower yourself back down.

Forward bends: Not all Yoga exercises are difficult. Try Forward bends as a way to increase the circulation in your legs, and strengthens the lower back and the spine. To do this exercise, sit with your legs wide apart in front of you and gently bring your head down to one of your knees. Hold this for a minute or two and then move on to the next knee. Easy as pie.

Quick Tips

Here are some quick tips to get the most out of your Yoga and Meditation sessions

1. **Do it first thing in the morning.**

Meditating early in the morning when you are refreshed from a good nights sleep makes it much easier to get into a relaxed state. This habit can also energize you for a peaceful day ahead at work. Give it a try and see.

2. To clear your mind, follow the lights behind your eyes.

This technique is a great one for clearing your mind of distracting thoughts. You know the lights that you see behind your eyelids when you close them? Imagine that you are hunting them and these lights are easily spooked by sound. Instead of the distracting thoughts, focus on silently 'following' the lights into your mind. This technique is also quote good for insomnia.

3. Start with quick meditations at first

Meditation is a skill that improves like any other skills, through patience and practice. If longer meditations are a problem, don't worry, you'll work up to them. Try quick 2 minute meditations and work your way up to the longer ones. You'll get there.

4. Don't worry that you are doing it wrong.

Everyone thinks that they are doing it wrong the first time. If you still can't proceed without worry, try obtaining some guided meditations online. Guided meditations are exactly what they sound like, meditation sessions where an experienced teacher walks you through the visualizations, generally with the accompaniment of pleasant music. These can be a good way to get started if you are still worried but relax. Everyone thinks they are doing it wrong at first.

5. Find a community.

With social media, you are never truly alone. Better, finding communities that share your interest can be a snap. Check your Facebook or other social media groups which you subscribe to and even meet if the group is local. You'll be trading books and advice in no time.

6. Explore yourself.

Meditation is about achieving a higher sense of self-awareness. If you notice particular patterns of thought during deeper meditations take some time to contemplate them. You can learn many powerful things about yourself, you need only to listen.

7. Stretch.

Stretching exercises before your Yoga session can help to keep you healthy as you learn some of the more challenging positions. Always take the time to stretch in the morning first as forgetting this can result in a lesson that you will certainly remember but only want to learn once.

8. Evolve your breathing exercises.

Alternate your breathing exercises to see what results come of them. Proper breathing is important for meditation and good for a number of other things as well, such as pain management and efficient exercise. Pay attention if a particular breathing pattern seems to get you relaxed more quickly.

9. Scented candles.

Scented candles improve the atmosphere when doing your meditation exercises and can help you get into a contemplative state much more quickly. Which brings us to our final tip.

10. Notice the sounds and scents around you.

When meditating take in the sounds and scents all around you. Are there birds outside? Does the house still smell like breakfast? Contemplating these smells and sounds can lead to a deep meditative state, so take advantage.

Next we would like to introduce you to a powerful Kundalini breathing technique known as the 'Breath of Fire'.

The Breath of Fire

This exercise is practiced worldwide by many practitioners of Kundalini and does many things for you, with its efficacy growing over time as you use it more and more. As it is one of the more strenuous techniques we recommend that you spend only short intervals of time practicing first and above all, be patient. Time invested in learning these techniques is time well-spent and should be used to learn the techniques WELL. It should be noted at this time that this exercise should not be done if you are pregnant or suffer from high blood pressure. Like other exercises that can strain the body you will want to use your best judgment.

So what exactly is the Breath of Fire?

The Breath of Fire is a Kundalini pranayama, or breathing technique. It provides a number of benefits, including:

- Strengthening the circulation of your blood for clearing out detrimental toxins.
- Strengthening the lungs - This exercise can help you breathe stronger and more clearly as it cleanses your body.

- Pain relieving - A number of breathing exercises are good for pain relief and this is one of them. If the exercise is difficult at first, don't worry, this is something that you will build up to.
- Stimulating the Sacral Chakra while strengthening the abdomen.
- Stimulating the mind from increased oxygen flow to your brain.

To perform the Breath of Fire, perform the following steps:

1. Sit up straight, don't slouch, form is important.

2. Begin breathing in a relaxed manner through your nose.

3. Here comes the tricky part. Push in your abdomen during the inhale. Push it out during the exhale. Note that this takes time to master, so if you only try this exercise for 30 seconds at a time, it's fine.

4. Shorten the breaths, inhaling and exhaling in the proscribed manner as quickly as possible. With practice, you can shorten and lengthen the breaths.

6. After about 30 seconds of of the breathing exercise, return your breathing to normal. Notice how your body feels energized? Some people report goosebumps (completely normal with this exercise).

7. Continue with the exercise, giving yourself normal breathing breaks. The intervals of time will increase and you will find that you can do more 'sets' of this form of breathing with increasing time between breaks. Don't overdo it or push yourself and be sure to take a rest before getting up whenever you are practicing more strenuous breathing exercises such as this technique.

Try to practice this Kundalini technique at least once a week and you'll notice your endurance growing. As we've mentioned previously, this exercise also strengthens the abdomen, so practice can also help you start looking good as you start getting more powerful in your meditations. If you find that this or other some of the other exercises might benefit from visual example, consider your local Yoga community or your personal computer or laptop at home. A number of videos and other media are present on YouTube and many, many Yoga sites that can helps with that extra bit of information that you might require with a particular pose, meditation, or exercise.

Conclusion

Together we have journeyed through many a subject. We have learned Chakras together. We have discussed the coiling energy of Kundalini, the Serpent energy, and empowered you with the basics of breathing and meditation.

They say that if you give a man or woman a fish that they will eat for a day, but we have taught you how to fish for yourself. Cultivate what you have learned and you can 'eat' for a lifetime. If friends ridicule you, keep them at a distance. There should never be ridicule for someone seeking to find their personal truths and what you have learned is the culmination of over 3000 years of study. We've showed you only the basics, bits and pieces, but the journey ahead of you will show you so much more. So as they say, 'keep the naysayers at bay', learn what you can and grow in wisdom and understanding. You know what is right for you and no one else in your life is going to seek, take, and ensure your happiness.

Be sure to practice your poses, your Mantras, and various Chakra meditations. This is not something that is going to happen overnight, you will need a little self-discipline to make sure that you keep on-track as you learn the Chakras and your Serpent Energies more intimately. Incorporate meditative self-contemplation in order to better understand yourself. Incorporate Yoga into your life to raise Kundalini energy while you are strengthening your mind and body. Incorporate the colors of the Chakras into your life to better cultivate their energies. Everything you need to get started and well on your path is here.

We thank you for spending time with us to take the very first steps and on the long road before you. We wish you only the best in your journey.

Know and understand the Serpent power, know your Chakra centers of energy.

Know them and more importantly, know yourself.

Namaste.

Manuscript 2

Reiki Healing: A Masterclass

The Step-by-Step, Comprehensive Guide to Master Reiki & Healing Meditation for Beginners

Siya Ishani

© **Copyright 2019 - All rights reserved.**

The content contained within this book may not be reproduced, duplicated or transmitted without direct written permission from the author or the publisher.

Under no circumstances will any blame or legal responsibility be held against the publisher, or author, for any damages, reparation, or monetary loss due to the information contained within this book. Either directly or indirectly.

Legal Notice:

This book is copyright protected. This book is only for personal use. You can't amend, distribute, sell, use, quote or paraphrase any part, or the content within this book, without the consent of the author or publisher.

Disclaimer Notice:

Please note the information contained within this document is for educational and entertainment purposes only. All effort has been executed to present accurate, up to date, and reliable, complete information. No warranties of any kind are declared or implied. Readers acknowledge that the author isn't engaging in the rendering of legal, financial, medical or professional advice. The content within this book has been derived from various sources.

Please consult a licensed professional before attempting any techniques outlined in this book.

By reading this document, the reader agrees that under no circumstances is the author responsible for any losses, direct or indirect, which are incurred as a result of the use of information contained within this document, including, but not limited to, — errors, omissions, or inaccuracies.

Table of Contents

Introduction

CHAPTER 1 - Why try our approach to Reiki Healing?

CHAPTER 2 - Reiki History Primer

CHAPTER 3 - Reiki Basics - The Principles, How it works, and Meridians

CHAPTER 4 - Reiki Self-Healing Exercises

CHAPTER 5 - The Three Pillars and Reiki Healing for Others

CHAPTER 6 - Chakra points and Reiki: Are they compatible?

CHAPTER 7 - Incorporating Chakra Points into Reiki Healing

CHAPTER 8 - Reiki and Kundalini: Are they compatible?

CHAPTER 9 - Using Reiki in conjunction with Kundalini

CHAPTER 10 - Reiki -Full 12 Meridian Healing

CHAPTER 11 - Healing stones to incorporate into Reiki and Chakra Healings

Conclusion

Introduction

"Every house is built on a foundation, and the foundation of your body is your life force. If the Chi is unhealthy it will affect the physical aspects of your life and thus our Reiki system is the key to unlock this impediment to your progress."

Are you suffering? Have your Doctors, Psychologists, and Psychiatrists tried to talk or medicate you to "health". Have you seen little or no results? Well, that's not surprising...

In today's hectic world, more and more people are suffering with seemingly ever-increasing health issues. Issues with weight loss, or weight gain are great examples of our problem with modern medicine.

We meticulously plan out our diets and follow through with our exercise and see poor results. The math says that we've eaten this many calories, and burned that many calories, so we should be loosing weight, and yet we don't achieve our goals.

You might also have a significant other that you're having problems with, or that you'd just like to be closer to. Perhaps you've tried picnics in the park, dance lessons, and more, but yet you still both find yourself arguing at the over little things that shouldn't really matter.

An unhealthy Chi can lead to an unhealthy relationship. Reiki, especially when done by both members of a couple, can provide a tranquility of spirit that allows both members to relax and grow together in harmony, instead of growing slowly apart in discord.

Ailments such as arthritis, migraines, carpal tunnel and others can be alleviated with the proper allocation of Reiki healing in conjunction with your current medical regimen. Often pain is simply a symptom of an energy imbalance in the body, and Reiki is designed to address this very situation specifically.

Reiki Healing can also help with chronic fatigue or insomnia by addressing the inconsistencies in your energies that you might not even be consciously aware of. Do you notice periods where your physical energy waxes or wanes for no reason that you can attribute to diet or environment? Then the Reiki system laid out here could be the answer.

If you've been suffering from panic attacks or other forms of anxiety, and nothing the doctors have prescribed or the psychologists have had you 'talk out' seem to help, then consider adding Reiki to your medical regimen. Doctors don't generally subscribe to the fact that a disharmony of the life force can be just as important as medications or psychobabble. This leads to a treatment of *symptoms* while ignoring the *source*. Reiki can bring a balance to your treatment and may be the only thing that you need, but you won't know until you try it for yourself.

As we progress through this book, we'll discuss how and why this system WORKS, as well as giving you the tools, so that you learn and practice Reiki healing from the comfort of your own home. As you learn to manipulate your life-energies you'll soon find that you can have the results that medical science has failed to provide time and time again.

It's all about what you know.

There are a number of reasons that you've come to Reiki and we hope not to disappoint. Simply pursue this knowledge with patience, learn what you read, practice what you learn, and soon let what you've learned become what you truly know. The results that arise will make it worth your while.

Let's continue to Chapter 1 and begin preparing you for the bright future ahead!

Chapter 1 - Why try our approach to Reiki Healing?

You probably know that Reiki is an energy-healing system but do you know how it works?

The Chinese have a word called 'Chi', very similar to 'Prana' or 'life force' to the Hindus, and it's fundamental to the way that Reiki healing works. Chi is present in everything and pervades the universe. Think of it as personal energy resonating with the energy of the Universe.

Literally translating as 'air', like the air that you breathe in every day in order to sustain yourself. Believers in Chi, Prana, Auras and other concepts of life energy abound across the world and use this energy to their benefit. Not just practitioners looking for healing - many martial artists subscribe to the belief as well, using the energies to protect themselves or to improve the veracity of their attacks.

With Reiki, our concern is going to be utilizing the Chi for healing and harmony. As it travels through our body it employs body-highways known as meridians and knowing the location of these Meridians can empower you to heal many ailments quite quickly and quite successfully. We'll go into more about the Meridians and Reiki applications through them later.

In the Introduction we advised you of some issues that Reiki can assist you with. Here are a few more issues that Reiki can address

(Keep in mind, this is still just a taste of what you can learn to heal. Reiki can do all of these things, and more):

Reduction of stress levels in your life

Reiki healing creates not only harmony but a state of deep relaxation that can decrease stress factors in your life. Think about it in practical terms. Have you ever had to make a decision in an emergency? When you're relaxed then you're much more likely to make a sound, reasonable   judgment call then when you're panicked or over-stimulated due to stress.

Increase the body's ability to heal itself from harm

Reiki works with your Chi energy, which when balanced, is said to improve your self-healing factor. When the body's life force is healthy this effect is only natural. Add is a little exercise and you'll find your body performing at peak capacity.

Help in cleansing the body of the toxins that we ingest each and every day

We ingest a surprising amount of toxins from day to day, often in the form of chemical additives or preservatives in products that might not be as '100% natural' as advertised. Reiki improves circulation and the body's ability to shed toxins, thus improving your overall health.

Stimulating creativity for those who wish to express themselves artistically or otherwise

When your energies are balanced through Reiki, you'll find yourself more receptive to the inspirations of your surroundings. A healthy Chi leads to less distractions and in such a state of harmonic bliss you'll find yourself better able to create.

Bolstering the immune system to fend off or fight sickness

As the body's energy is balanced with Reiki healing, the immune system steadily grows more efficient. This can lead to your body producing more white blood cells and giving your immune system a much-needed boost for a healthier life.

Intrigued? You're in good company. A 2007 study indicates that 1.2 million people in the United States alone have taken the time to explore the benefits that Reiki can provide them. This demonstrates a general unhappiness that the medical community alone has been insufficient to address. Thus, other measures are quite obviously required.

You're in the right place!

Our approach can help you to address these issues and many, many more.

So, are you ready to get started?

Great!

First we are going to discuss a little of the history of Reiki and then we'll get you started on some healing basics. You'll then start building your Reiki-toolbox with some new and powerful techniques as we go.

Chapter 2 - Reiki History Primer

What's the history behind Reiki? Well, Reiki originally hails from Japan, the brainchild of a man named Mikao Usui.*

Mr. Usui, a lay Monk (a non-clerical monk, who takes local vows but wasn't ordained), Mikao was living in a time in Japan's history when a wide variety of spiritual practices were commonplace, with Buddhism, Shinto, and Taoist beliefs being the primary modes of spirituality.

In the early 1920's (reportedly 1922) Mikao would have a profound spiritual revelation that he'd spend the last 4 years of his life sharing with the world.

Usui Reiki was born.

While containing Reiki healing techniques, the mass of Mikao's teachings amounted to quite a bit more, with philosophies and insights not only from Japanese traditions but from ancient Chinese medicine as well. Excited about his spiritual discovery, Mikao Usui travelled the length and breadth of Japan to spread his revelations, bringing students into the fold who shared his enthusiasm for this new system of ancient wisdoms.

While he taught more than 2000 students before he died, he had appointed only 16 of these to be Reiki Masters. One of the Masters, a retired Naval officer by the name of Chujiro Hayashi, received Mikao's blessing to open a clinic in Tokyo. Having worked extensively with Usui, Chijuro desired to take the healing aspects from the main body of Usui's teachings and make them more accessible to the general public.

From this, he developed his own style of Reiki, keeping meticulous notes as the 16 Masters at his clinic worked, leading to data in regards to which hand positions were most favorable for treatment. He also began imparting healing elements of Chinese medicine, such as Meridians, and Hindu elements such as Chakra points into his practice.

Chijuro, like his mentor, began training masters as well, and one of them would be a Japanese-American by the name of Hawayo Takata.

Hawayo had herself been healed from a number of ailments through Reiki treatment and, as such, became a devoted student of Sensei Hayashi.

Eventually she'd bring Reiki to Hawaii in 1937.

Eventually, she'd bring Reiki to the mainland United States. During her life, she taught for 40 years before beginning the training of her own Reiki Masters, of which there were 22 at her time of death in 1980.

Modern Reiki has evolved but as it employs ancient wisdom at the core, much has stayed the same. While Takata's 22 Reiki Masters have spread her teachings and style, in this day and age a number of styles and combinations are practiced worldwide.

It just goes to show that Sensei Usui was on to something...

Chapter 3 - Reiki Basics - The Principles, How it works, and Meridians

The 5 Principles of Reiki

1. *Just for today, do not be angry*
2. *Just for today, do not worry*
3. *Just for today, be grateful*
4. *Just for today, work hard*
5. *Just for today, be kind to others.*

While much of Mikao Usui's teachings were excised by Chijuro in favor of promoting strictly the healing precepts of Reiki , much of Miikao's teachings still remain. The 5 precepts of Reiki are one of these principles. These are words to live by, elegant in their simplicity, let's take a moment to contemplate this wisdom.

1. Just for today, do not be angry.

We get angry over the slightest things. Things that sometimes don't even matter in an hour or two, except as 'water cooler' talk (and what a state of things, when we tell stories of someone cutting us off in traffic and how angry we got, as if two ugly things suddenly have more merit then the beauty in life.)

Take a day off from your anger.

Take today off from your anger. When you feel it coming up, contemplate something that made you laugh, or something profound like the birth of your child, or even just distract yourself by trying to describe the smells around you in a mental dialogue. Try this little experiment and at the end of the day ask yourself, 'Was my day better or worse without the anger?'. Just something to contemplate.

2. Just for today, do not worry.

Worry does very little for us and quite a lot of things against us. Increased stress levels raise our blood pressure. Too much worry can promote anxiety or rash decisions. Try to turn that energy, if only for today, into either preparation or fuel for a more productive day. Another good alternative is rest, as the Vikings used to say, 'If you spend all night worrying about the battle, then you'll be tired in the morning when you must fight it.'

3. Just for today, be grateful.

It's amazing how often we can forget the things that we've in lieu of complaining about the things that we want. A roof, enough food, employment - these are things that people across the world and even close to your home simply don't have. Is it really worth your sense of peace to create a bad day for yourself and others just because they left the onions off your sandwich at a restaurant or your friend gave you a Pepsi instead of a Coke?

You have your health and a full belly, you're already ahead of the game and from a practical standpoint, time spent feeling ungrateful is time you could be spending writing that bestselling novel, painting that new work everyone will marvel at, prototyping your genius invention, or planning that amazing small business. When you catch yourself (and sometimes it's easy to forget), stop yourself from being ungrateful. Try it, just for today.

4. Just for today, work hard.

One of life's little-known and oft forgotten pleasures and treasures is the feeling that you get from a job well-done. We get lost in our daily routine and after awhile it seems like we are running on autopilot. While you might feel tempted to just fly through the day like a robot, why not take the time, assert your will and your power of self, and show them just what you've got? Oddly enough, this simple precept gives you a way to break out of your routine while you're in the middle of experiencing it. Just for today, let it be your first day at work, give it your all and see how you feel when it's behind you. You may be pleasantly surprised.

5. Just for today, be kind to others.

Sometimes the world seems to move at the speed of light. We feel like we need to push ahead, streak past whatever is in our path, and get it all behind us. The problem with this is that it's an attitude towards time, rather than an attitude towards the world. When we push and rush we tend to find ourselves being rude to others. When we assume that every homeless person is simply out for a drink, then we sometimes consign good people to hunger while we starve our own souls in the process.

Slow down.

Today, be kind. Feed the birds. Give the dog an extra treat. Give the homeless guy some change. Offer your sibling the last pancake. There is an endless list of little things that you can do to be kinder and every little bit makes the universe that much better. Just for today, don't take, but give.

How it Works

Now that you've had a taste of the philosophy, let's get to the reason that you came here. You want to learn how to perform Reiki healing. So, we mentioned Chi earlier, that energy that's inside us and all around us. When it comes to the body, your Chi travels along paths inside it called Meridians. These Meridians help ensure the flow of Chi where it needs to go in your body. Think of them as 'Chi Superhighways'.

Now, when the Chi is blocked or otherwise imbalanced (too much Chi here, too little Chi there) then the problems start and the longer that it's harmony is imbalanced the worse it can get. Resulting in something as innocuous as a bad mood on a particular day and up to more serious conditions like bipolar disorder or even heart problems.

This is serious stuff, folks. Why do you think a culture as old as China still utilizes Meridians in acupuncture and other treatments?

People like to scoff but despite the progress of current medical science, these ancient concepts are obviously doing something for millions around the world that's actually working.

So, we've established that Chi needs to flow properly and that Meridians are the roads that it utilizes in your body, next we should logically talk about Meridians. These are going to seem complicated at first as you'll need to memorize, over time, the circuitous paths that they take through the body. As a homework assignment after you read the rest of this chapter, get a piece of poster board at the store, then do a Google search and copy diagrams of the Meridians so that you can make a collage of their locations. Hang it up in the house somewhere where you'll see it often. You'll be going through exercises in the following chapter that will teach you exactly what paths the meridians take but creating a creative visual aid can help immensely as you begin your path as a Reiki Healer.

If you're ready, let's discuss Meridians. Applying this knowledge will take a little practice, but once you understand the pathways that the Chi energy takes through your body, then you'll understand how to better manipulate these energies within the framework of Reiki.

If you're ready, let's continue to the individual healings of the 12 Meridians.

The 12 Major Meridians

While the Meridians are identified by particular parts of the body, that doesn't mean that they only govern that part of the body. It's a little more complicated than that but we're going to cut through the haze for you, cut it down into bite-sized chunks, and ensure that you get the understanding that you require. After all, we aren't writing an encyclopedia entry here, our job is to give you just what you need to get started and get practicing.

1. **Kidneys**- Producing bone and marrow through a chemical called EPO, kidneys also store sexual energy and regulate the development of sexual organs. You'll notice that we mention Asthma and Tinnitus as well, this is because these issues can be due to deficient kidney Chi. Be sure to take care of this meridian.

Location: Starting from the sole of your foot, this Meridian then travels up the inside of your leg, then to your abdomen and terminating just below the clavicle.

Physical effects:

- Tinnitus
- Asthma
- Backache
- Urinary issues

Emotional effects: This Meridian controls your force of will. A blockage or imbalance in this Meridian can cause a feeling that you're lacking control in life, unable to effect change no matter how hard you try.

2. **Spleen**- The Spleen performs a number of important functions. Regulating your blood flow, for one, and also regulating your digestion. As it's an important part in the transport of nutrients and their accompanying Chi, it also regulates your muscle density.

Location: This Meridian starts just outside of your big toe, coming up the inside of your leg to your thigh. It continues to your abdomen and up further, passing the outside of the nipple to your second rib, where it starts down again and terminates at the 6th intercostal space (6th space in your ribs, counting down from your head)

Physical effects:

- Abdominal issues (constipation, diarrhea, bloated feelings)
- Poor muscle density
- Prolapsed internal organs
- Chronic fatigue

Emotional Effects: Blockage or imbalance in this Meridian can cause you to feel mentally slow or absent-minded.

3. **Liver**- The Liver governs the menstruation and the female reproductive cycle. It's also responsible for your tendons and ligaments. Most importantly, this organ is among the most important for storing and circulating Chi throughout your body.

Location: Starting inside your large toe (underneath the nail), this Meridian runs up the inner leg, up to your thigh, and then travels to the outside of your abdomen on the way to its terminus, which is your sternum.

Physical effects:

- Stiff joints
- Menstrual issues
- Vertigo
- Jaundice
- Blurry vision or dry eyes
- Headaches

Emotional Effects: Blockage of this Meridian can lead to a number of negative effects, such as anger, depression, and limited range of emotional expression due to an 'emotional lockdown'.

4. **Heart**- As the steward of your veins, arteries, and capillaries, the heart is immeasurably important to your physical health. It's also quite important to your mental health, as well. See below.

Location: This Meridian is a bit less complex to trace than the others. It starts in your arm pit, travelling down your inner arm and terminating at the fingernail on your pinky (smallest) finger.

Physical effects:

- Insomnia
- Dizziness
- Chest Pains
- Shallow breathing
- Cold sweats and hot flashes
- Bipolar disorder (from prolonged blockage or imbalance)
- Tachycardia/Heart Palpitations

Emotional Effects: This Meridian relates to your happiness. As such, it can cause a number of psychological issues if blocked, such as bipolar disorder, anxiety, depression, and obsessive-compulsive disorder. It also directly associates with an aspect of Chi called 'Shen', which is essentially our spirit and mental health... the presence that we exude. A number of issues can occur with imbalance, as you see, so be sure to perform healings upon this Meridian should you suspect that something is amiss.

5. **Lungs-** Your lungs regulate not only your respiration but also your intake of Chi energy.

Location: Starting at the first intercostal space between your ribs (the space between your first and second rib, starting underneath your head), this meridian goes up the shoulder and down the front of your arm, terminating at the fingernail of your thumb.

Physical effects:

- Problems with your sense of smell
- Upper body sweating and inflammation
- Coughing and congestion
- Skin conditions

Emotional Effects: A number of effects can occur when this Meridian is out of balance, such as depression, intolerance, false pride, contempt, or even as an inability to process grief.

6. **Pericardium-** The membrane that encloses your heart. Aside from the governance of its Meridian, the Pericardium holds importance as an energy center of the body that you can draw upon for healings. This is because the Pericardium not only protects the heart but it dissipates excess energy from the heart which you can draw into your palm to distribute to areas that need it.

Location: Beginning on the outside of the nipple, this Meridian travels from here up your shoulder and then down the front of your arm, terminating at the fingernail of your middle-finger.

Physical effects:

- Stomach issues
- Heart issues
- Chest pains

Emotional Effects: Imbalance or blockage in the Pericardium Meridian can cause issues with personal expression/communication with others, as well as paranoia, and phobias.

7. **Gall Bladder**- Storing and excreting excess bile, problems with this organ's Meridian can some serious health and emotional issues as listed below.

Location: This Meridian takes a long path through the body, starting at the outer corner of your eye, going inside your head and downward, and then down the front of your shoulder. From here it enters inside of your abdomen and then out again, travelling further down on the outer side of your leg where it terminates at your fourth toenail.

Physical effects:

- Yellowish tinge to the tongue or skin
- Liver pain
- Feeling bloated

Emotional Effects: Imbalance or blockage of the Gall Bladder Meridian can cause feelings of rage, excessive pride, and an overly judgmental attitude.

8. **Bladder** - Responsible for excreting liquid waste from the body.

Location: This Meridian starts at the inner corner of your eye, where it then goes over the top of your head, moving down your back and legs until it terminates at the toenail of your pinky (smallest toe).

Physical effects:

- Back Pain
- Stiffness in your shoulders and neck
- All diseases of the Urinary system
- Chronic headaches

Emotional Effects: Blockage or imbalance of the Bladder Meridian can cause issues with emotional expression, a 'hair-trigger' temper, restlessness, and extreme frustration.

9. **Stomach-** The stomach digests your daily meals and extracts Chi from them, distributing it to your spleen and intestines.

Location: This Meridian begins just under the center of your eye, going down the face to the very edge of your jaw, and then back up to your forehead. From here, it travels down to your throat, continuing to the front of your abdomen, down the front of your leg, terminating at the nail of your second toe.

Physical effects:

- Digestive issues

Emotional Effects: Effects that can occur from blockage or imbalance of this Meridian include feeling unaccepted, nervousness, constant worry, and an increased urge to criticize others.

10. **Small Intestine-** Distributing nutrients throughout the body, as well as Chi extracted from digested food, Blockage of the Small intestines can result in one or a number of ailments listed below.

Location: This meridian starts at the fingernail of your pinky finger, going up along the back of your arm to your shoulder. It travels down your shoulder and then back up to the neck, moving finally to your ear.

Physical effects:

- Acne
- Neuralgia
- Abdominal pain
- Lymph node swelling
- Weakness in your legs
- Always feeling cold
- Stomach distention
- Nerve pain

Emotional Effects: Negative emotional impacts from blockage or imbalance in this Meridian can include feeling unappreciated, indecisiveness, nervousness, and constant feelings of discouragement.

11. **Large Intestine-** The large intestine removes water from waste matter, absorbing it and excreting the solids.

Location: This Meridian starts at the fingernail of your index finger. From here, it goes up your arm, behind your shoulder, and then up to your face, terminating at your nose.

Physical effects:

- All abdominal pains are connected with this Meridian.

Emotional Effects: Blockage or imbalance in this Meridian can result in an Inability to hold on or to let go of people in your life.

12. **Triple Warmer (your body's thermostat)-** This isn't actually an organ, rather it's a concept of Chinese medicine. You might call it your metabolism, but that's over-simplifying things. The Triple Warmer regulates body temperature, metabolism, and liquids. As such, virtually every imbalance that relates to an organ is going to relate to the Triple Warmer as well. The Triple Warmer, dissected, looks like this:

- *Upper Warmer-* Governs the upper part of your body, including your head, neck, heart, lungs, and your chest.
- *Middle Warmer-* The area between your navel and your chest, including the liver (special, see below), spleen, and the stomach
- *Lower Warmer-* Also governs the liver, your bladder, and the kidneys.

As you can see, this one is a bit more complicated at first but to keep it simple, be sure to include this in the healing of any Meridian, as it's always going to be part of an imbalance.

Location: This Meridian starts at the nail of your ring-finger, going up your forearm and continuing over the back of your shoulder. From here it continues around your ear and terminates at your eyebrow.

Physical effects:

- All

Emotional Effects: As the Triple Warmer covers all of the body, then consider any emotional dissonance to require a healing of the Triple Warmer as well as the associated other Meridians.

The Three Extraordinary Meridians

Now that we've discussed the 12 Major Meridians, we need to tell you about the Extraordinary Meridians. While there are 8 of them, only 3 will be used in Reiki healing. These 3 act like spiritual batteries, storing Chi power that can be circulated through the body as needed. We won't go into too much detail on each at this time, as they're a little advanced but we wanted to include this information so that would have knowledge of these further Meridians to explore. The 3 Extraordinary Meridians are as follows:

1. **Ren Mai** -'The Conception Meridian'

Location: Beginning inside your mouth on the very tip of your tongue, this Meridian follows a path down the front of the body until it's terminus at your perineum.

Function: This Meridian governs all of your Yin Meridians.

2. **Du Mai** - 'The Governing Meridian'

Location: This Meridian begins at your coccyx, where it then travels up the spine until it terminates at a spot just behind your teeth.

Function: This Meridian governs all of your Yang Meridians. It's also responsible for protective/defensive aspects of your Chi.

3. **Dai Mai** - 'The Girdle Meridian'

Location: Running parallel with your kidneys and your navel, this Meridian is so named because it wraps around the body like a girdle.

Function: This Meridian governs your sense of balance.

Yin and Yang Meridians

- *Spleen and Stomach*
- *Lungs and Large Intestine*
- *Liver and Gall Bladder*
- *Kidneys and Bladder*
- *Heart and Small Intestine*
- *Pericardium and Triple Warmer*

Above is the listing of Meridian pairings for the Yin and the Yang. Your Chi requires these forces to be balanced and your Meridians are paired in relation to each other and their aspects. With Reiki healings and acupuncture, when an imbalance occurs then the associated organ of the pair must be healed as well, for it's also out of harmony with its paired Meridian. Thus, if you're performing a Lungs Meridian healing, you'll also wish to perform a Large Intestine healing, in order to restore their harmony so that Chi may flow unimpeded. Sound complicated? Don't worry, we've got you covered, as you'll see in the exercises. You'll find it's not difficult, only new. Let's continue to the next chapter, 'Reiki Healing Exercises' and we'll show you.

Chapter 4 - Reiki Self-Healing Exercises

Finally, down to the nitty-gritty! We've given you a little bit of a foundation to get you ready for this moment. It's time to learn how to perform your first Reiki healings. These healings may be done just once for an ailment or, better yet, multiple times. Issues that took awhile to develop can take longer to address, so just keep in mind that sometimes you'll want to do many treatments to ensure proper healing.

Before we get started with exercises, we should take a moment to advise you in regards to the importance of proper breathing. Proper breathing techniques can help you with a number of things, including dealing with pain, narrowing your focus when you need to be sharp, and relaxing enough to reach a proper meditative state. Is it complicated? Nope, or at least, it doesn't have to be. There are advanced techniques, of course, that can take quite a bit of time to learn. All you need to get started, however, is a simple exercise that we'll detail for you now. Learn it, practice it, know it. It's primitive but it will get you where you need to go!

So, if you're ready, let's outline the steps for your first breathing exercise.

Breathing exercise

> *1. Sit somewhere comfortable for practice. This way you don't have any distractions. Once you're used to measured breathing then it becomes second nature, indeed, in times*

of stress you might find yourself automatically employing breathing techniques that you've mastered. Once you're comfortable let's move on.

2. Inhale slowly for a count of four.

3. Hold the breath slowly for a count of 4.

4. Exhale slowly for a count of 4.

That's it! Simple, but effective. You can try alternating your counts, for instance, inhaling for 4, holding for 4, exhaling for 3 to see how it makes you feel. Different combinations can produce different results.

Experiment with them to see what gets you feeling healthiest and most focused. It seems a simple tool at a glance but you might be surprised at the applications that you'll find.

Now that you know how to breathe properly, we're going to start you off with the Triple-Warmer healing, as this Meridian will need to be healed in conjunction with any other Meridians that you're treating. Due to its nature (regulation of body temperature, bodily fluids, and metabolism) the Triple Warmer is almost always going to be imbalanced when there is an imbalance with the other Meridians.

Getting into the habit of doing this can make your healings more efficient. One note, if you like, record yourself reading the steps of these healings and play it with a little music while you practice. Keep the music instrumental so that it's not distracting. This is a great way to learn a healing if you like a hands-free immersion rather than sitting and memorizing from the book. Typically Reiki healing will involve particular hand placements, and we'll go into those later, but this method allows you to perform Reiki and to commit the Meridians properly to memory.

Reiki Healing for each of the 12 Meridians

Triple Warmer

> 1. Begin your breathing exercises, getting nice and relaxed.
>
> 2. Visualize your own Chi flaring around you as a bright white light surrounding you and inside of you. Try to get a feel for how it flows through your body. Do you feel the blockage that's present? If not, don't worry, this will come with time.
>
> 3. Place your hand, palm open and fingers spread slightly at the place over your Pericardium. As we mentioned before, it's the membrane enclosing your heart that drains excess energy , so we are going to take advantage of this. With your Chi energized through visualization, start pulling the excess energy into your palm. See it gathering as a ball of light, almost too bright to look into.
>
> 4. We are going to now move the ball of light as we move our hand over the Meridian. It should be noted, many practitioners will just hold a hand over the head or chest and trace the Meridians through visualization. You can certainly do that if you like but it's good practice to practice tracing the Meridians at the beginning to learn them. You might find you actually prefer moving your

hand, however, as it feels quite graceful. That said, Start by placing your open palm over the nail of the ring finger. Visualize the Meridian like an electrical cable made of its own white light. Move your hand with the ball of light and see it crackling with white Chi energy as you bring it up your arm to your shoulder, moving it over and behind your shoulder slowly as you bring it up to the top of your ear and stop at your eyebrow. See the ball of light getting smaller as it transfers the energy, finally disappearing at the terminus of the Meridian. You may notice warmth or tingling when you do this, don't worry, this happens sometimes as you become more advanced and it's a good thing.

5. Next, we must consider the Yin and the Yang relationship for this Meridian. The Triple Warmer is considered to be the Yang aspect of a pairing with its Yin component, the Pericardium. To ensure the balance, take more energy from your Pericardium to make another ball of Chi light and move your palm over the Pericardium meridian. This movement will be very close to the opposite of the Triple Warmer meridian. Move your open palm to be just over the outside of your nipple. Move your hand slowly up to the shoulder and then down your arm, stopping at the nail of the Middle finger. As before, see the ball of light slowly diminishing as it feeds the Meridian, charging it and destroying imbalance and blockages.

6. Move your palm over the Meridian patterns that you just traced in this healing, focusing to see if you still feel any blockage or imbalance, or if they feel energized now to you. It may take practice to develop the sensitivity to this

so be patient. Some people are lucky enough to be able to do this naturally but most people will need a little practice. Don't worry if you're one of the latter because you'll develop the sensitivity soon enough.

7. If you sense no blockage or if you're still learning your sensitivity and not sure, then relax your breathing and consider your first healing done. Do you feel differently after this? Invest in a notebook or a blank book to journal your healings and progress, it's a good way to learn and to document your steps along the Reiki path.

Next, we are going to go over a healing for the kidneys.

Kidneys

1. Begin your breathing exercises, reaching the inner calm where you're ready to undertake this working.

2. Visualize your own Chi flaring around and inside you as your awareness expands from your measured breaths.

3. Place your hand , palm open and fingers spread slightly, over your Pericardium. Draw forth the Chi energy into your palm, a white ball of healing light.

4. Move your palm, the ball of light travelling with it, through the path of the Kidney Meridian. You'll start at the sole of your foot, moving the light up the inside of your leg. Bring it up further still to your abdomen and higher still, to the clavicle bone. See the line of the Meridian as clearly as you can in your mind, now crackling with the healing energy that you collected from the Pericardium.

> 5. The kidneys possess a Yin aspect and the Yang of the kidneys is the Bladder. Draw another ball of light from your Pericardium and let's empower the Bladder Meridian. Move your palm and Chi sphere up to your face, to the inner corner of your eye. moving it up and over the top of your head and then down your back. Continue down your leg until you reach the foot and the ball dwindles to nothing at the nail of your smallest toe. As before, visualize the Meridian line as you commit it to memory through practice. See it winding through its path, filling with power as you send healing energy and purge blockage and imbalance.
>
> 6. Draw another healing sphere of Chi from your Pericardium and perform the Triple Warmer Healing to ensure that the organs you've healed and the body's regulator are all in harmony.
>
> 7. Trace the associated Meridians to feel for blockage. Feeling anything yet? Don't worry, keep practicing.
>
> 8. If you sense no blockage or are still learning your Meridians, feel free to consider this healing practice complete.

Practice, practice, practice!

Let's continue now to learn a healing for the Spleen.

Spleen

> 1. Begin your breathing exercises, as previously.

2. As your consciousness expands, visualize your Chi, blazing brightly.

3. Place your hand, palm open and fingers slightly spread, over your Pericardium. Take the excess energy coming from the Pericardium into your hand, forming it into a ball of light.

4. Move your palm and Chi light-sphere down to your foot, to the outer edge of your big toe. Move it from here slowly up your leg and further up, to the thigh. Move it higher still, up the abdomen and bring it up to the outside of your nipple until you get to your second rib. Move it down again to the terminus. the 6th intercostal space of the ribs (the intercostal space is the space between your ribs). As with the previous healings, see the Meridian lines as you're tracing them. Watch them filling with the energy as the sphere slowly diminishes.

5. The Spleen is considered to be the Yin in it's pairing with the Yang of the Stomach. That said, let's balance the Yin and the Yang to ensure these organs function in harmony. Draw an energy sphere of Chi from your Pericardium again and move your hand up to your face, holding it just over the center of your eye. Don't worry, this light is very good for you. Begin moving it down your face to the edge of your jaw, then up to your forehead. Move your palm of light slowly and to your abdomen, where you'll take it down the front of your leg to your foot and the Meridian's terminus, your second toenail. Visualize the stomach Meridian shining brightly now, free from blockage and imbalance and complimenting it's other half of the Yin and the Yang, the Spleen.

6. Perform the Triple Warmer healing to ensure that we are being thorough.

7. Now that we've performed the healing, trace the Meridians with your palm again, both for practice and to see if you can feel them flowing with unimpeded Chi.

8. If you sense no blockage, consider the healing a success.

Let's move on to our next candidate, the Liver.

Liver

1. Begin your breathing exercises so that you're in the proper mindset.

2. Begin visualization of the Chi energy around you, the same energy that pervades you and everything in the universe. See it as a bright light surrounding and filling you.

3. Place your hand, palm open and fingers slightly outstretched, over the Pericardium. Draw the needed energy into an orb so that it's ready to be redistributed.

4. Move your hand with the healing Chi down to your foot. Starting at your big toe (visualize the line starting under the nail), trace your open palm up your inner leg and bring it up to the thig. Move it further up along the outside of your abdomen, watching as it feeds the Liver Meridian with white light crackling like electricity. Continue up to the sternum and you've completed the circuit. See the entire Meridian glowing clean and bright with the energy that you've placed there and commit as much of it as you can to memory. Soon you'll know it like the back of your hand.

5. The Liver is considered to be the Yin aspect of its Yin/Yang pairing with the Gall Bladder. Move your and back to your Pericardium and draw forth more Chi. Feel it as a warmth in your hand and hear it crackling. We'll need a lot of energy, as this Meridian takes a long path through the body. Move your hand to the outer corner of your eye. Let the orb loose and see it going inside your head and downward towards the front of your shoulder. Catch it with your palm and bring it slowly down your abdomen, letting it loose again to go inside, as you move your palm downwards. See the orb coming back into your hand, smaller now as it expends its energies. Next, you'll move it down the outer side of your leg and take it gently to its terminus, the nail of your fourth toe. This one is a little more complicated but you'll learn it. Towards this end, try to see it glowing brightly in your mind's eye, filled with the energy that you fed into it. Your Gall Bladder and Liver Meridians are now working, once again, in youthful harmony.

6. Perform the Triple Warmer healing to rule out any imbalances that may have been caused by the Liver and Gall Bladder Meridians when they were in disharmony.

7. Trace the Meridians that we've just worked with via your open palm. See if you can feel the harmonies of the Meridians that you've just worked so intimately with.

8. If you sense no blockage, let's move on.

Heart

1. Begin with your breathing exercises to get centered.

2. Open your perception and see your Chi power, burning brightly.

3. Place your hand over the Pericardium, with your palm open and your fingers spread slightly. Draw upon the excess Chi that your body is shedding and shape it into an orb. Take a moment to enjoy the wonder of its brilliance. Like a boxful of puppies or kittens, a baby's smile, ice cream on a hot summers day...this is the stuff of life.

4. Move the Chi energy in your open hand to your armpit. Now move it slowly down your inner-arm and take it gently you the nail of your smallest finger. Visualize the Meridian glowing fiercely from the energy you just requisitioned for it. Commit it to memory and let's continue to balance it's counterpart.

5. The Heart Meridian is the Yin of its Yin and Yang pairing with the Small Intestine. To heal the Small Intestine and restore full harmony to the twain, move your hand to your Pericardium, palm open and fingers spread slightly, and draw fresh energy into it and shape it as an orb in your mind. Move your hand to the opposite hand, holding it over the fingernail of your smallest finger. Move it upwards, over the back of your arm to your shoulder, the orb of Chi light becoming smaller as you progress. Bring it down from your shoulder and then back up to the throat. From here, bring tiny orb up to your ear where the last of the energy you collected will be absorbed in the Meridian.

Note the Meridian, now free of blockage and empowered, blazing with light, and commit what you can to memory.

6. Perform the Triple Warmer to ensure thoroughness of this Health-working.

7. Trace all of the Meridians that we've worked with on this healing to see what the energies feel like to you. Do you still feel a blockage or do they feel like running-rivers of energy?

8. If you sense no blockage, let's continue.

Lungs

1. Start your breathing exercises in preparation for manipulation of your Chi.

2. See your Chi, around and within you, shining brighter than any searchlight.

3. Place your hand, palm open and fingers slightly spread, over your Pericardium so that we may collect the excess Chi energy. Draw it into your hand, a blazing sphere of healing light.

4. Move your hand upwards towards the top of your ribcage, stopping at the beginning of the Meridian. This will be the first intercostal space or, simply put, the first space between your first two ribs. Slowly move the Chi-light up your shoulder and let it move down the front of your arm, the ball decreasing in size as the energy flows into the Meridian. Continue down the front of your arm until you reach your thumbnail where the tiny orb will at last deplete it's energy. Take a moment to enjoy the sight of this Meridian, brightly flaring and free of blockage before we continue to its Yin and Yang counterpart.

5. The Lungs are considered the Yin i the Yin and Yang pairing that exists with its counterpart, the Large Intestine. Let's move our open-palmed hand back to the Pericardium and once more collect healing Chi energy. Gather up your sphere of white light and bring it with your hand down to the fingernail of your index finger. From here, bring it up your arm to the back of your shoulder, and as the sphere of light dwindles, bring it up furhter to your face and it's terminus, your nostrils.

6. Perform the Triple Warmer healing to ensure that this is also in balance and to ensure efficacy of this working.

7. Trace the Meridians with your hand to see what you feel. By now it's likely that you're developing sensitivity to these energies. Good job. Soon you'll be ready for other techniques as well.

8. If you sense no blockage, let's move on and don't forget, some healings may take multiple sessions so don't be afraid to perform this or other healings multiple times in a week.

Now we'll move on to our friend, that 'electric company' of spare Chi, the Pericardium.

Pericardium

1. Begin your breathing exercises, as always. Don't neglect proper breathing, it's much easier to enter the mental state needed for these workings.

2. See your Chi in all its glory, blazing around and filling you. We are ready to go..

3. Place your hand, palm open and fingers slightly spread, over your pericardium. As we are doing a healing for the Pericardium, as you attempt to draw energy, meantally pull at some of the Chi that's surrounding you as well. You're one with the Universe, so drawing this energy is simply borrowing from yourself. It replenishes.

4. Move your open hand and hold it over the space just outside of your nipple, taking it slowly up your shoulder and then down the front of your arm. See the ball of light diminishing and feel any blockages exploding in the healing light of your Chi and you move the dwindling orb to this Meridian's terminus, the fingernail of your middle finger. Take a moment to admire this Meridian of light that serves the body as a pathway for your Chi. Soon you'll know this pathway by heart.

5. As we are familiar with the Yin Yang pairing already (the Pericardium pairs with the Triple Warmer), perform the Triple Warmer Healing to continue.

6. Traces the Meridians of both the Pericardium and the Triple warmer to see what you feel. Do they feel blocked still? Harmonious? They should feel healthy and restored after the working.

7. If you sense no blockage, we may continue to the Gall Bladder.

Gall Bladder

1. Begin your breathing exercises to prepare.

2. With each time you practice, it becomes easier and easier to see the Chi around you. Take a moment to congratulate yourself for your patience and perseverance. Bask in your Chi a moment and let's continue.

3. Place your hand, palm open and fingers slightly spread, over your Pericardium. Draw the excess Chi and feel it filling your hand with warmth and healing power.

4. We described the healing Meridian-path of the Gall bladder when we discussed the Liver, however, as it's one of the more complicated Meridians to memorize, we'll list it again for you.

"Move your hand to the outer corner of your eye. Let the orb loose and see it going inside your head and downward towards the front of your shoulder. Catch it with your palm and bring it slowly down your abdomen, letting it loose again to go inside, as you move your palm downwards. See the orb coming back into your hand, smaller now as it expends its energies. Next, you'll move it down the outer side of your leg and take it gently to its terminus, the nail of your fourth toe."

5. Move your hand over your Pericardium and collect more healing light from your Chi. Direct the orb with your hand over the Liver Meridian from earlier in this chapter.

6. Perform the Triple Warmer healing.

7. Trace the associated Meridians to feel for blockage or imbalance.

8. If you're satisfied with what you sense from the Meridians, it's time to move on.

Bladder

1. Begin your breathing exercises to get properly relaxed.

2. Visualize your Chi, powerful and blazing around and within you, ready for this working.

3. Place your hand, palm open and fingers slightly spread, over your Pericardium. Collect the excess Chi energy into your palm in a ball of white light.

4. Move your hand up to your face to the inner corner of your eye, where it then goes over the top of your head. As the Chi-light slowly diminishes while empowering the Meridian, move it down your back and legs until it the Meridian terminates at the toenail of your pinky (smallest toe) and fully absorbs the Chi sphere.

5. As we learned from a previous healing in this chapter, the Bladder is the Yang of the Yin and Yang coupling it has with the Kidneys. Collect more energy from your

Pericardium and perform step 4 from the Kidneys healing to empower the Kidney Meridian for balance.

6. Perform the Triple Warmer healing to ensure balance.

7. Check the Meridians from this healing with your hand and your growing sense for energies.

8. If you sense no blockage, we can move on to our next healing.

Stomach

1. Begin your breathing exercises to get centered.

2. Once centered, open your awareness to see your Chi energy around you and inside you. We are ready to continue.

3. Place your hand, palm open and fingers spread lightly, over your pericardium. Pull the excess Chi energy from it and let it form into a ball of blazing light.

4. Move your hand up to your face, just under the center of your eye. Move the Chi-sphere in your hand down to the edge of your jaw, then up to your forehead. From here, move your hand down your throat slowly as the energy from the sphere enters the Stomach Meridian. Continue down the front of your abdomen, down the front of your leg until you arrive at its terminus, your second toe.

5. The Stomach Meridian is the Yang of the Yin and Yang pairing it enjoys with it's Yin, your Spleen. Draw energy once more from your Pericardium and heal the Spleen

Meridian (only performing step 4 from the healing listed earlier in this chapter)

6. Perform the Triple Warmer Healing in order to ensure that the previous blockage has caused no imbalance.

7. Trace the Meridians associated with this healing to ensure that the flow of Chi through these Meridians is healthy and unblocked.

8. If you sense no blockage, consider the healing a success.

Don't worry, we only have two more to go. We hope that you've taken our advice from earlier and created a journal for your progress. This is often the best way to get a good idea how you're advancing and also to keep track of how often that you're practicing. Reiki is a rewarding path for a long and healthy life. That said, without further ado, Let's move to the first of the last two healings in this chapter, your Small Intestine.

Small Intestine

1. Begin your breathing exercises and clear your mind so that you'll be receptive to your Chi,

2. Visualize your own Chi, enveloping you from head to toe in brightest of lights, pure life and divine bliss.

3. Place your hand, palm open and fingers slightly spread, over your pericardium. Pull the excess Chi energy into your hand in a ball of blazing white.

4. Move your palm and Chi sphere to your opposite hand, bringing the light to the start of the Small Intestine

Meridian, your pinky (smallest) finger. Move the sphere up the Meridian, which is up the back of your arm to your shoulder. See the orb diminishing in size as you continue up to the neck and to the Meridian terminus at your ear. See the Meridian crackling with energy. From practice with the previous Healings it's likely quite familiar to you by now, almost an old friend. Let's continue.

5. The Small Intestine is the Yang component of its pairing with the Yin Heart. Reaching over to your Pericardium, gather more excess Chi light into an orb and use that orb to heal the Meridian for your Heart to balance the two Meridians. Employ only step 4 from the Heart Meridian Healing.

6. Perform the Triple Warmer healing in order to ensure balance.

7. Check the Meridians with you hand, open palm and fingers slightly spread, tracing their pathways to feel their energies. Do they feel more balanced?

8. If you sense no blockage, we are ready to continue to the last of the healings from this chapter for you to practice. Good job.

Large Intestine

1. Begin your breathing exercises so that you may be receptive to your Chi energies.

2. Visualize your Chi, bright and powerful from your practice and previous healings.

3. Place your hand , palm open and fingers slightly spread, over the Pericardium. Draw up the energy that we'll need into a healing orb and let's continue.

4. Move your hand and healing Chi to your opposite hand, targeting the fingernail of your index finger. Move the healing sphere up your arm, watching as it gets smaller as it expends energy in destroying blockage and empowering this Meridian. Continue moving the healing light up and behind your shoulder and then up to your face, depleting the orb as it terminates at your nostrils.

5. The Large Intestine is the Yang to its Yin of your Lungs. Move your hand to your Pericardium and draw another Chi healing sphere's worth of energy and then use it to trace and heal the Lungs Meridian. Heal the Meridian only, don't perform the full Lungs healing.

6. Perform the Triple Warmer healing in order to ensure proper function now that the Large Intestine and Lung Meridians are again in harmony. i

7. Use your sensitivity, beoming more honed with your practicing to check the integrity of the Meridians that you just healed.

If you're happy with the results of this healing, then you're ready to move on.

This concludes our chapter on Reiki Self-Healing exercises. Next we are going to discuss the Three Pillars. a foundational Reiki working set that Mikao Usui developed both for use before healings or even as part of your daily routine. We're going to follow that with a Tradition-based Reiki healing where you'll learn the traditional hand-placements now that you've enough knowledge of Meridians to utilize them. This is where it all comes together.

Chapter 5 - The Three Pillars and Reiki Healing for Others

The Three Pillars of Reiki

Aside from the 5 Principles of Reiki, Usui taught the Three Pillars as a form of foundational practice for Reiki. These meditations should be performed before each session (some like to perform the Gassho meditation every morning) and the guidance portions will help to hone your intuition into something you can trust easily.

So, to begin, we'll tell you about each Pillar and then we'll provide information on how to observe the Pillars before you perform a Reiki Healing.

1. **Gassho** - Translating as 'Two hands coming together', Gassho is many things, among them a moment of cleansing followed by what amounts to a spiritual statement of intent. Lastly, projecting the feeling of gratitude to the collective conscious for the healing that you're about to perform.

2. **Reiji-Ho** - Translating roughly as 'the indication of Reiki power', Reiji-Ho is essentially asking for your hands to be guided. This aids in your goal of becoming intuitive about what Meridians are out of balance with little to no effort.

3. **Chiryo -** Translated as 'Treatment', this part is all about action rather than meditation. HHaving performed Gassho and Reiji-Ho, the practitioner begins the laying of hands in places where it's required. At first, you'll be utilizing the standard order of hand arrangements as you learn the body placements but eventually, through Chiryo, you'll develop a sense for where to place them.

So how does one invoke these Pillars? Well, with Chiryo it's, as we said, simply practice. For the first two you'll access their energies in this fashion:

Gassho invocation

> *1. Find somewhere comfortable to sit (you can do this standing if you like, whatever you're most comfortable with).*
>
> *2. Begin your breathing exercises to get in the proper frame of mind.*
>
> *3. Close your eyes and bring your hands in front of you, closed in a 'prayer' position. Press your fingers close together and focus your attention to the tip of your middle fingers. Recite the 5 Principles of Reiki:*

> *Just for today, do not be angry*
>
> *Just for today, do not worry*
>
> *Just for today, be grateful*
>
> *Just for today, work hard*
>
> *Just for today, be kind to others.*

4. When you're finished, project your feelings of gratitude to the Universe, to the collective consciousness... and you're done.

Next we'll continue to the guidance portion of your pre-healing routine. Invocation of Reiji-Ho will help your intuition immensely and the effect is cumulative, as you'll soon see.

Reiji-Ho Invocation

The Reiji-Ho invocation is done in 3 small parts.

- **Part 1:** With your hands positioned as before when you performed Gassho, close your eyes and ask for the Reiki power to flow through you. Visualize energies of all colors coming from all directions into you, brightening your Chi like a star. You're now empowered for your healings.
- **Part 2:** Ask the Universe for the issue to be healed. Ask for their recovery on all, even the unexpected levels.
- **Part 3:** Ask the Universe and the Reiki power to guide your hands, bringing them where they're needed so that your patient may be healed wholly.

Now you may continue to Chiryo, where you practice your Reiki healing hand positions. In time, you won't have to do all of them, just the ones that are needed.

Let's continue now to your first Tradition-based Reiki healing. It will be much easier than you're expecting. Now that you know the Meridians, all you need for Reiki healing is the proper mindset, the Pillars, and your hard-earned knowledge of the Meridians.

Excited? Then let's continue.

Tradition-based Reiki Healing

In traditional Japanese Reiki, there are hand placements that are used for healing the Meridians. While typically you don't touch someone when you're doing the healing, you can lay hands upon them (with consent), hold your hands slightly over them in the correct locations, or place the persons own hands in the correct position with yours over them (good for the areas that are a little more private). Now that you've a working knowledge of the Meridians that you'll be working with you're ready for a tradition based healing. This requires no special ritual, so to speak. Basic placement over the affected areas and focus on the proper flowing of the Chi is all that's required. That said, a little explanation as you work can go a long way with your patient so that they understand exactly what you're doing. For future healings, simple hand placement in the correct areas combined with your knowledge of Meridians is all that's required. You can talk about your day with the patient as normal. Chi goes where it's meant to go by nature, all it needs sometimes is a little Reiki nudge.

Here are the steps that you can use to provide a tradition based Reiki healing for another person. Use these steps to learn the hand positions and soon you'll be ready to perform these healings on your own.

Steps for Reiki Healing

1. Have the recipient of the healing lay down flat on their back somewhere comfortable and easy to reach. When you become adept at Reiki, you might consider purchasing an old hospital bed or a massage table for your healings as these are the proper height for a Reiki session.

2. Place both open palms over your patient's pericardium. Let them know that it's function is expelling excess Chi and that you're going to be drawing that forth to redistribute throughout the body as needed. Let them know also that this treatment is completely non- invasive, involving only your knowledge of the flowing of Chi and the proper placement of your hands to nudge it along, as their body does the rest, and that the patient may feel free to have a nice chat with you as things continue without fear of disrupting the energies.

3. Place your hands in the **First Position**.

Location: Face, covering the eyes.

- *With the First position you'll be standing behind your patient, hands cupped slightly above their eyes. Don't touch, just hold the hands above (depending on your personal style and the patient's comfort level) Alternately, you may place the patients hands over their eyes and your own above them if that's more desirable to the one that you're healing.*

4. Hold your hands in place and feel the flow of Chi throughout the Meridians. See Chi flowing through them, destroying obstacles in its path so that the life energy flows freely along each Meridian, as it should.

5. Next we'll assume the **Second Position.**

Location: Top of the recipient's head.

- Bring your hands back slightly so that the inside of your wrists are touching at the top of the head and your hands are placed so there is one on each side, with your fingertips almost touching their ears.

6. Hold your hands in place and feel the energy flow of Chi, travelling through the body, empowered and stimulated to flow by your treatment. Keep your hands in place for as long as it feels necessary before moving on to the next position

7. Move your hands into the **Third Position**.

Location: The back of the Recipient's head.

- Ask your patient to lift their head slightly. For this position, touching is more convenient for you but this will, of course, be up to the recipient of this healing and their own personal comfort levels. If they're okay with touching, then hold both hands together underneath their head, supporting it comfortably. If they're not comfortable with touch, simply assume the same position with your hands and request they hold their head up for a moment until this part of the healing is complete.

8. With the Chi energy that you're holding in your hands the flow of Chi should be restored shortly and we may continue to the next position.

9. Now we'll place our hands in the **Fourth Position**.

Location: Covering Cheeks and chin and wrists almost touching the ears.

- The Fourth position involves cupping the patient's face from behind, thumbs should be level with the cheeks, fingertips touching or almost touching underneath the chin, and the heels of your hands almost touching their ears. This is another Position where the ability to touch is favorable but let's keep everything within the patients comfort zone.

10. Take a moment holding your hands in the Fourth position, gently coaxing the Chi energy to go it's natural path. Feel the warmth as the current of Chi assumes it's natural flow.

11. You're ready to place your hands in the **Fifth Position**.

Location: Throat, and the Center of your Patient's chest.

- You'll place your right hand, slightly curled over the patient's neck. Place your left hand over the center of the chest, next to the Heart.

12. Leave your hands in this position as more of the excess Chi restores the proper flow of energy.

13. Moving beside your patient, place your hands in the **Sixth Position**.

Location: Center of chest/upper ribcage.

- Place your left hand over the left side of the ribcage, just under the breast level, and place your right hand over the right side of the ribcage.

14. Take a moment to focus on the energies flowing properly. Visualize the Meridians closest to this area as you empower them with your hand placement and the excess Chi. ,

15. You're ready now to place your hands in the **Seventh Position**.

Location: Your patient's Solar Plexus.

- Move your both of your hands down to the Solar Plexus/'Belly' area. This is just above the Navel.

16. Move your hands down further into the **Eight Position**.

Location: Your patient's Pelvic bones.

- Moving both hands down further still and pulling them apart slightly so that one hand is over each Pelvic bone, you've now assumed the Eighth Position.

17. Let the excess Chi drain further, coaxing the natural flow of Chi energy through the recipients body. When you feel that the energy is flowing at peak level, move on to the next position.

18. When you're ready, have the patient roll over onto their stomach. Now you may place your hands in the **Ninth Position**.

Location: Shoulder blades of your patient.

- Place your hands as before but this time on the shoulder blades, with your left hand over the left shoulder blade and your right hand over the right shoulder blade.

19. Feel the energy flow going from constricted to slightly widened, then from slightly widened to completely unobstructed. Once the Chi flow has been restored here from your hand placement we are ready to move on to the next.

20. Moving your hands down we are ready to stop them in the **Tenth Position**.

Location: The middle of your patient's back.

- For this position we are simply moving our hands slowly down until they're hovering over the central portion of the back.

21. Keeping your hands in place and visualizing the Meridian lines, observe as the Chi energy resumes a healthy flow.

22. Now we are ready to move the hands further down into the **Eleventh Position.**

Location: your patient's lower back.

- Moving further down, keeping your hands covering the left and right sides, move them over the lower back and stop, holding them in place.

23. Hold your hands in place until the energy flow of Chi feels healthy and productive.

24. Now we may move on to the **Twelfth Position**.

Location: Just above the tailbone.

- Move your hands down and hold over the area just above the tailbone (definitely no touching with permission.).

25. Hold your hands in place until you feel that any blockages have been erased and then we are ready to move on.

26. Move your hands down to the legs for the **Thirteenth Position**.

Location: Behind the knees and at the base of the ankles

- Place one hand over the space behind the knee and one hand over the lower ankle.

27. Hold your hands here and allow the flow of Chi to reassert itself while you visualize Chi energy flowing to the terminus points of the Meridians that terminate in your feet.

28. Move your hands to the final placements, the **Fourteenth Position**.

Location: The soles of your patient's feet.

- Reaching over or simply stepping in front of the patient, place your hands over but not touching the soles of their feet.

29. Take a moment again to feel the energy from the Meridians that terminate at this point.

30. The healing is complete. Ask your patient how they're feeling. Most will report feeling relaxed and refreshed, their Chi flowed restored to its proper, unobstructed flows.

Now you know the healings, the daily rites. What you do with them is up to you. In the next chapter we'll expand your knowledge, what you do with it, for good or ill, is up to you. Hopefully you won't go all 'dark Reiki' on us after all of this time, practice a little patience and you'll soon be a healer of merit. Keep what you've learned close, focus your morale, and above all: heal.

Chapter 6 - Chakra points and Reiki: Are they compatible?

Now that you've learned some basic Reiki healing we would like to introduce you to another system that can be used in conjunction with your current techniques to enhance and strengthen your results.

We're talking about Chakra Points.

So, what exactly are Chakra Points and are they really compatible with Reiki?

Chakra Points are a system of Hindu derivation that have a rather interesting scope. Based on writings called the 'Vedas', written between 1000 and 1500 years B.C., the actual word 'Chakra' translates out as 'wheel'. This is based on the belief that around you and inside of you is your life force, a spinning energy that turns the 7 Chakra-wheels inside of your body. If one of them is turning too fast or too slowly then it can lead to imbalances that must be addressed to be healthy both spiritually and physically.

My, my... this sounds a little familiar, no?

As you can see, these systems have quite a little bit in common. As such, incorporating Chakra points into your Reiki healing is a powerful way to enhance your current techniques, much like a blacksmith makes an alloy of two metals that turns out to be stronger than either one would be alone. Is hybridizing the system truly more efficient? Well, that's for you to decide.

We just provide you with the toolbox, what you decide to use and make from these tools is truly up to you.

Now that we've piqued your curiosity, we'd like to give you a brief introduction to Chakra points in this chapter, followed by another chapter with exercises so that you can practice incorporating the two systems to see if it's to your liking. Now, Chakras are basically 7 points of energy centers, which start at the base of your spine, climbing straight up to the top of your head. These Chakras are fed energy from channels in the body called 'Nadis'. Now, while Reiki has the Meridians, Nadis are similar in function but different in number. While there are 12 Meridians that you've memorized and used often by now, there are 72,000 Nadis.

Before you run screaming, no, we are not going to have you memorize them. You won't need to know them to use what we are about to teach you. Just your Reiki basics and the information about Chakra points that we are about to provide. So, without further ado:

Chakra Points - A Basic Primer

Before we continue, it should be noted that we are going to simplify using Chakras within the framework of your Reiki healing. There are colors associated with the 7 Chakra points are actually the 7 colors of the rainbow and as this isn't only easier to remember but very, very practical for effective visuals in meditations, we are going to use the color names as the primary focus for your Chakra manipulation. 'Proper' names will be included within the description of each so that you're educated in the Sanskrit name and the most common names of the Chakras but for what we are doing, the color focus is just as effective and much easier to remember.

Remember, this is a guide for just starting out. Should you decide you wish to learn more about integrating Chakras and Reiki at a later date there is much reference material out there for you to explore. We are just here to get you started. Now, here are the 7 Chakras so that you may familiarize yourself with them before we begin practical applications in the next chapter.

The 7 Chakra Points and their Healing Applications

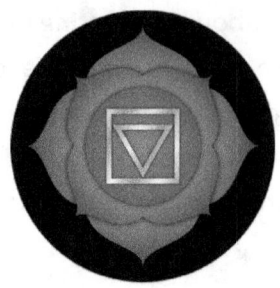

1. Red Chakra - Muladhara - Root Chakra

Muladhara in Sanskrit means 'Root' or 'Support', and as such is also known as the Root Chakra. Located at the base of the spine, This Red Chakra rules over your survival instincts. Fight or Flight, Self-Preservation.. It's the sovereign center of survival. As a results of this influence the Red Chakra also affects your reliance on material possessions to feel secure and accomplished at home. Sexually, it governs the urge for procreation in how it relates to you feeling secure in home and family.

Healing Associations

- Your lower back
- Your legs
- Your Hips
- Your coccyx
- Your sexual organs (if Male)

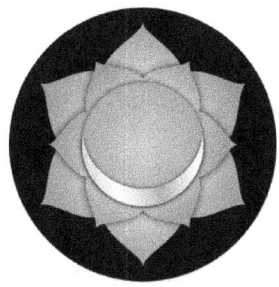

2. Orange Chakra - Svadhishthana -Sacral Chakra

Commonly known as the Sacral Chakra , the name of this Chakra in Sanskrit translates as 'Sweetness'. So what is its purpose and where is it? Located below the navel, the Orange Chakra is quite important for how we interface with life. The Orange Chakra governs how we process experiences in life and how we connect with others. Basically put, the health of this Chakra determines how we deal with triumph and tragedy and our very sense of self. From another emotional aspect, a healthy Orange Chakra allows us to utilize our inner strength for ourselves as well as others. Think of it as sort of a 'radio station of the self' in this aspect, if the Chakra is healthy then you and other can hear your music and announcements loud and proud, whereas a blockage makes the signal scratchy and hard to understand completely.

Healing Associations

- Your large intestine
- Your colon
- Your bladder
- Your sexual organs (if Female)

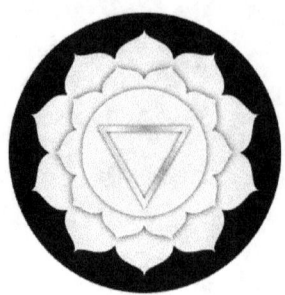

3. Yellow Chakra - Manipura - Solar Plexus Chakra

It's Sanskrit name translating as 'Lustrous Gem', the Yellow Chakra is located at your stomach. Where the Orange Chakra broadcasts your self-power like a radio station, the Yellow Chakra is the actual seat of said power. This Chakra is strongly tied to both your personal and professional life. To the personal portion of your life, it's your ability to understand yourself as you truly are. A blocked Yellow Chakra can lead to self-delusion, so deal with blockages quickly if you suspect there might be one here. From a personal and professional level, the Yellow Chakra determines how much you can communicate who you're to the world at large. It also reflects your personal abilities and skills. Meditations on this Chakra can be quite useful when acquiring new skills, so be sure pay attention to its health.

Healing Associations

- Your gall Bladder
- Your stomach
- Your kidneys
- Your liver
- Your pancreas

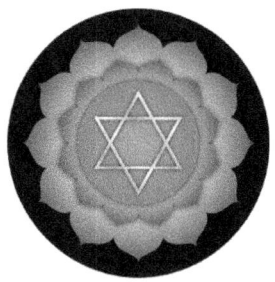

4. Green Chakra - Anahata - Heart Chakra

The translation in Sanskrit for the Green Chakra is fitting with it's 'Heart' appellation. It's name translates to 'Unhurt, Unstruck, and Unbeaten'. Located at the center of the chest, the Green Chakra governs how much we are able to love ourselves and others. As such, like the Orange Chakra, it can determine how we process our experience and the lessons of life. After all, questions such as 'Do I love myself' and 'Do others love me?' have a profound effect on whether we take a fall as a lesson or a punishment.

Healing Associations

- Your heart (of course)
- Your breasts
- Your lungs
- Your arms
- Your upper back

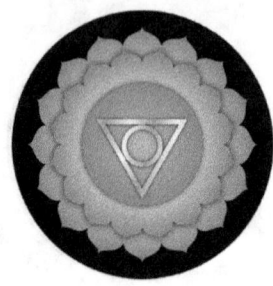

5. Blue Chakra - Vishuddha - Throat Chakra

In Sanskrit, 'Vishuddha' means 'Purification', and in governance aspects the Blue Chakra rules communication with the self and with others but in a very particularly way. Stay with us on this.

The Blue Chakra governs another very important aspect of life, *your creativity*.

The poets, writers, and artists of the world all require that the Blue Chakra remains unblocked, as it directly affects their ability to take a concept or abstraction and make it into something solid that the world may understand and enjoy. This Chakra is located at the base of your throat.

Healing Associations

- Your mouth
- Your ears
- Your thyroid
- Your larynx
- Your throat
- Your neck

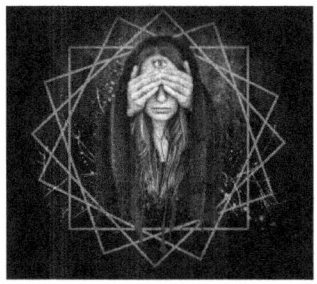

6. Indigo Chakra – Ajna - Third Eye Chakra

While the common name, 'Third Eye Chakra' makes you think this is only for spiritual perception, the Sanskrit name is much more accurate when describing it's function. Translating as 'To perceive', the Indigo Chakra governs spiritual awareness, yes, but it also governs your ability to think logically, to perceive what is true in an unclouded fashion. The Indigo Chakra let's you take immediate problems or perceptions and then make a conscious decision to 'pull-back' and see things from a birds-eye perspective. Interpreting the bigger picture, if you'll. The Indigo Chakra is, of course, located just above the eyes in the center of the brow.

Healing Associations

- Your pineal gland
- Your lymph nodes
- Your brain
- Your sinuses
- Your eyes
- Your endocrine system

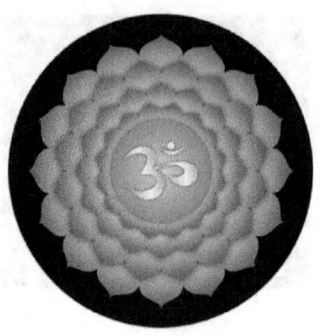

7. Violet Chakra - Sahasrara - Crown Chakra

'Thousandfold' is its name is Sanskrit, the Violet Charka is the seat of your Spiritual power. Located at the top of your head, this Chakra governs your connection with all things spiritual as well as your awareness of your connections with the universe. Foresight is also affected by the Violet Chakra, as knowing your place in the bigger picture gives you a stronger chance to accurately predict or know your future.

Healing Associations

- Your joints
- Your spine
- Your cervical vertebrae

Now that we've learned some basics about the Chakra system, let's continue to some exercises where we can incorporate this with your current Reiki skill set. The results from the pairing of two powerful systems can be extraordinary, as you're soon to find out. So, when you're ready, let's continue to our next chapter, 'Incorporating Chakra Points into Reiki Healing'.

Chapter 7 - Incorporating Chakra Points into Reiki Healing

Now that you've had some grounding in the basics of Chakra points, it's time to put that information to some use. As an exercise, try each first the way that they're currently listed and then try adding Meridian practices that you've already learned. See what is most efficacious for you. Once we've completed these, we are going to continue to learn a little about another compatible energy called 'Kundalini', which can help to power up your healings and comes with the added bonus of increasing awareness. These are all just building blocks that we are stacking upon the Reiki foundation that you've already constructed. Extra tools in your toolbox. Let's continue with practical applications of the Chakra information that you've learned and we can go from there.

Chakra and Reiki Healing Meditations

Here is your list of meditations. Above all, be sure to practice what you learn here so that you can incorporate this information into your healing toolbox. This will be a little different from what you're used to. Let's begin.

Red Chakra and Reiki healing meditation

Affected body parts:

- Your lower back

- Your legs
- Your Hips
- Your coccyx
- Your sexual organs (if Male)

1. Find yourself someone comfortable to lay or to sit down. You might be here awhile so make sure it's a comfortable place, free of distractions. Draw power from your Pericardium when you're ready.

2. Place your hand, palm open, fingers spread just over your Red Chakra point (the base of your spine). It can be in front of you or behind you, but front is easier for comfort.

3. Close your eyes and begin your breathing exercises , as discussed in our Reiki meditation chapter.

4. Once you're relaxed, clear your mind and begin focusing on visualizing the Chi around your body. See it as a white light that surrounds you and pervades you.

5. Begin focusing this energy into your Red Chakra, which you'll see as a glowing red sphere. Say it's Sanskrit name, 'Muladhara'. As you say the name, see energy flowing in pulses, like flickering electricity. With each recitation, see the Chakra glowing a brighter and brighter red.

6. When the light is as its fullest, Look upon the Chi with your Red Chakra, see how they integrate in harmony. Contemplate this for a moment and we are ready to continue.

7. Begin reciting 'Health to my _____' for each associated body part.

Example:

'Health to my lower back'

'Health to my legs'.

8. With each recitation, see the Chi energy flowing from you into the Chakra, which in turn brightens and sends energy to the body part on which you're focused.

9. When you've completed all of the body parts, slow your breathing and open your eyes.

That's it. Your first Reiki and Chakra meditation. Practice this so that you may better familiarize yourself with the healing location associated with the Red Chakra. When you're comfortable, we may continue to the Orange Chakra.

Orange Chakra and Reiki healing meditation

Affected body parts:

- Your large intestine
- Your colon
- Your bladder
- Your sexual organs (if Female)

1. Go back to your comfortable spot or find yourself a new one. Note, Nature is good for this too, as long as you've a pretty place where you won't be disturbed. Feel free to make a dedicated place or to mix it up a little, whatever makes you most comfortable. Draw power from your Pericardium when you're ready.

2. Place your hand, palm open and fingers spread over the spot just below your navel. This is the location of your Orange Chakra.

3. Close your eyes and begin your breathing, as we did in the previous exercise.

4. Once relaxed, visualize your Chi burning brightly around you. Focus this energy to your hand.

5. Now we'll being focusing energy into your Orange Chakra, which you'll see as a glowing orange sphere. Begin repetitions of its Sanskrit name, 'Svadhishthana', and with each repetition see the Chi flowing from your hand into the Orange Chakra. which responds with blazes of orange fire until it's burning brightly.

6. Now that your Chi and your orange Chakra are both blazing and in harmony, take a moment of contemplation to see if any insights come on how these energies play together. It's important always to pause for contemplation as there are always new things to learn about the interplays of these energies.

7. Begin reciting as before, 'Health to my _____' for each associated body part.

8. See the Chi energy becoming Orange Chakra energy and direct that energy to each body part. Visualize them as best you can. In very powerful meditations, sometimes you'll feel a tingling or a warmth. Don't worry, this is normal.

9. When you're done all of the associated body parts, relax your breathing and open your eyes.

Remember, practice makes perfect, and learning the Chakra associations with healing is our goal, so memorize but above all, practice these meditations.

Yellow Chakra and Reiki healing meditation

Affected body parts:

- Your gall Bladder
- Your stomach
- Your kidneys
- Your liver
- Your pancreas

1. Find your favorite meditation spot and get comfortable. Feel free to add music to your meditations if you like, sometimes it helps for deeper and fuller meditations. Just nothing too distracting, we want the focus to be within and not without.

2. Place your hand, palm open and fingers spread over your Yellow Chakra, which is conveniently located at your stomach.

3. Close your eyes and begin the measured breathing portion of your meditations. Be sure to get good and relaxed for the best results, we don't want any distractions that come with a stressed and agitated mind.

4. Let your awareness spread slowly from your center until it encompasses a few feet outside of the body. See your Chi, white light blazing and mysterious, at one with yourself and yet at one with the entire universe.

5. Properly humbled and yet also empowered, let's send some of this energy into the Yellow Chakra. See it as a glowing yellow sphere, like a perfect orb of clear Citrine filled with its own inner light. Begin repeating it's Sanskrit name, 'Manipura'. With each repetition see the white Chi light pouring into the sphere which is filling with golden light, as if with water. Once it's full, see it shining brightly and clear as glass.

6. Take a moment to contemplate the beauty of this interplay of energies. Ponder that the Yellow Chakra is the Chi and the Chi is the Chakra. It's a reflection of oneness with the self and the Chi energy of the Universe around you.

7. Recite, 'Health to my _____' for each associated body part.

8. As recite this, see light coming from your Yellow Chakra as if it were focused by a magnifying glass, like the 'water' of Chi power that you filled it with has enabled the Chakra a heightened focus. Feel a healing warmth as it touches each body part.

9. Once you've completed this, relax your breathing and open your eyes. You're done.

Work, sleep, rinse and repeat. You'll find that you learn these meditations quite quickly, just be sure to make time on your schedule or better yet, practice one daily before work.

Green Chakra and Reiki healing meditation

Affected body parts:

- Your heart
- Your breasts
- Your lungs
- Your arms
- Your upper back

1. Get nestled in your meditation cove, comfortable and ready for this working.

2. Place your hand, palm open and fingers spread over your Green Chakra, which is located in your central chest area.

3. Close your eyes and relax. Begin your breathing exercises.

4. Open your awareness and see the Chi flowing around in and in you. Bask for a moment in the energy of the life of all things in the Universe.

5. Collect the energy around you and focus it into your hand as you visualize the green Chakra orb inside you. Say it's name, 'Anahata', repeating it like a chant as your Chi flows into the Chakra which, in turn, then fills organically as if plants of energy were growing upward and twining together until they join as one bright and shining whole.

6. Observe your proper contemplations as always. Just as you relate to the world with different aspects, each Chakra relates with your Chi in its own fashion. Observe, learn, and listen to the silence for a truth or two. We are not in a hurry.

7. Recite, 'Health to my _____' for each associated body part.

8. With each recitation, see your Chi empowering the Green Chakra which in turn reaches out vines of green energy, wrapping the focus of each recitation in healing warmth, suggesting growth and regeneration.

9. Once you've addressed each of the body parts we've listed for the Green Chakra, relax your breathing and open your eyes anew.

Your Green Chakra is now empowered and the healing is in place. Take advantage and spend some time with someone dear, you'll find yourself better able to feel and communicate. Give it a try.

Blue Chakra and Reiki healing meditation

Affected body parts:

- Your mouth
- Your ears
- Your thyroid
- Your larynx
- Your throat
- Your neck

1. Find your meditation nook and sit down comfortably.

2. Place your hand, palm open and fingers spread over your Blue Chakra point. This one is located at the base of your throat.

3. Close your eyes and begin your breathing exercises.

4. As you become more and more relaxes begin to see your Chi flowing around you. If it doesn't seem bright enough around you, feel free to pull from the Universe to brighten it. You're one with the Universe so you're only borrowing from yourself.

5. Visualize a bright blue sphere underneath your hand. Say the proper name of the Blue Chakra, 'Vishuddha', and begin repeating it as a chant. See your Chi energy encircling and filling the sphere with blue light, starting from the edges and circling slowly as it fills the empty center.

6. Observe the interplay of the energies now that both your Chi and your Blue Chakra are in focus. Do you notice anything special in how they interact? You might consider keeping an insight journal for those moments of enlightenment that you wish to keep.

7. Recite, 'Health to my _____' for each associated body part.

8. With each repetition of 'Vishuddha', see your Chi energy empowering the blue sphere and bathing the body part that you're focusing upon in sapphire light. Feel a tingle as if from a cool wind on each, as if each has become healthy and antiseptic.

9. Once each body part has been addressed, let your breathing relax and open your eyes.

Don't forget to practice this often. You may find yourself especially creative after this exercise, do some writing, a little bit of art... take advantage.

Indigo Chakra and Reiki healing meditation

Affected body parts:

- Your pineal gland
- Your lymph nodes
- Your brain
- Your sinuses
- Your eyes
- Your endocrine system

1. You know the drill. Get comfortable and receptive to some deep workings. Now we are going to learn a Reiki healing that inorporates the Indigo Chakra. Let's continue.

2. Place your hand, palm open and fingers spread over your Indigo Chakra, which is located on your forehead, just above and between your eyes.

3. Close your eyes and begin your breathing exercises. Make sure that you're quite relaxed before continueing.

4. Visualize an Indigo sphere just under your hand opening slightly, like a sleepy eye as your Chi fills your vision, all around you and more brilliant than you've seen it previously. Take a moment of contemplation of this. Development of the Indigo Chakra can make you more sensitive to energies.

5. Say the name of this Chakra, 'Ajna', and begin repeating it in a chant. See the light of your blazing Chi flowing from your hand into the eye. See the Indigo eye becoming a deeper shade of indigo with each Chi infusion, opening wider as well until you feel a deeper awareness flooding inside you.

6. Definitely take a moment of contemplation this time. See the energies around and inside you. At this moment you're likely more spiritually perceptive then you've ever been before, so it's best to take advantage.

7. Recite, 'Health to my _____' for each associated body part.

8. With each recitation, see the Chi energy flowing from your hand and directing the eye to gaze upon the body part where you wish it to focus. See the gaze as an indigo searchlight and

each body part becoming clearly sharper in perspective and healthier with each full gaze placed upon them.

9. Once each body part has been sent healing energies from your Chi empowering the Indigo Chakra, relax your breathing and open up your physical eyes.

This working may produce odd dreams or the occasional intuitions. From the logic aspects of this Chakra you might also find yourself a little better organized. Don't worry, this is normal, enjoy.

Violet Chakra and Reiki healing meditation

Affected body parts:

- Your joints
- Your spine
- Your cervical vertebrae

1. Let's prepare by going to our meditation zone. Put on your favorite meditation music if you like and let's prepare to do a Reiki healing with the Violet Chakra.

2. Place your hand, palm open and fingers spread over your Violet Chakra point. This one is located at the top of your head.

3. Close your eyes, begin your breathing exercises, and get nice and relaxed.

4. Become aware of your Chi around you, surrounding you and flowing through your body through the Meridians and the Chakras.

5. See the Chakra at tthe top of your head, a violet sphere glowing fiercely. Address it by its name, ' Sahasrara' and begin repeating the name slowly. As you repeat the name, see your Chi energy flowing into the Violet sphere, filling it with a crackling fog of energy which coalesces slowly into a shining purple brilliance.

6. Enjoy your moment of contemplation and ponder how the Chi around and inside you interacts with the seat of your spiritual conscience.

7. Recite, 'Health to my _____' for each associated body part.

8. With each recitation, see the Violet sphere growing brighter and brighter, with the outlines of a face sometimes appearing within. Your face. See the sphere, directed by Chi and your spirit, directing violet energy to each part of the body that you wish to send rejuvenation and healing to.

9. Once you've finished with each body part for this Chakra, relax and open your eyes. You're done.

This rounds off our sample healings to get you a little practice with using Reiki in conjunction with your Chakra points. As we've mentioned, practice, practice, practice. You'll be surprised at the benefits that can come from this understanding of the body's energies so keep up your studies and absorb this wisdom. You'll be happy that you did.

Chapter 8 - Reiki and Kundalini: Are they compatible?

Around 500 to 1500 years B.C., a Hindu text called the Upanishads makes mention of a path of spiritual enlightenment known as Kundalini. The root of its Sanskrit name, 'kundalin', translates out to 'circular', which reflects the visualization of the energy. Kundalini energy is spiritual energy that resides at the base of your spine at the Red Chakra, coiled around the spine like a snake. As such, it's often referred to as 'The Serpent Power'.

Sound familiar? In Greek legend, there was a healing staff known as the Rod of Asclepius. The Caduceus, similar in design but with two snakes is the one you're probably more familiar with, however, due to its eminence as a symbol of healing adopted by Health organizations in North America.

It's interesting that such symbols of power are cross-cultural.

The Serpent power, said to rise up from the Red Chakra and stretching up to the Purple Chakra when a spiritual awakening has been achieved (and this is a good time to remind you that Mikao Usui had a spiritual awakening), you might think that this energy has very little to do with Reiki, which is primarily a healing system. In actuality, there are quite a few areas where Kundalini practice can't only have relevance, but where it can strengthen particular healing efforts and give us yet another useful tool in the growing toolbox of aspiring Reiki Healers.

For arguments sake, here are a few points in which Reiki and Kundalini coincide:

- Reiki involves laying the hands upon certain points in order to balance Chi. Chakras, a system we discussed before is similar, where health is reliant on the distribution of 'Prana', or life-energy. Kundalini incorporates Chakras heavily in it's system.
- Reiki requires you to unblock the Meridians so that Chi may flow. For spiritual awakening, Kundalini requires Sushumna, the central channel, as well as a number of Chakras to be unblocked before it may rise.
- Both teach principles of letting go of hate, compassion, and gratitude.
- Both disciplines possess powerful methods of healing the body and mind

These are just a few, of course. What matters most for us is the healing aspect. Medical doctors don't turn down new gear just because they're unfamiliar with it, if it can enhance their ability to heal.

In the next chapter we are going to introduce some exercises that you can try in order to determine whether Kundalini has a place in your own style or Reiki or not. You should be warned. As Kundalini is also geared towards spiritual awakening, should you begin getting headaches or having odd dreams then don't worry, these are just a few of the signs that you might be in for a spiritual awakening. If this occurs, spend a little more time with your Chakra works and perhaps invest in a little Kundalini research to help push it along. After all, even though healing is our primary goal, a little enlightenment never hurts. Let's continue to the next chapter and begin our exercises.

Chapter 9 - Using Reiki in conjunction with Kundalini

Now that we've given you a little foundation on Kundalini concepts and history it's time to incorporate a little training with a popular Kundalini medium. Mantras. Mantras are sacred words that are used for a number of reasons... protection, enlightenment, or in this case, healing.

We've gathered a collection of Mantras that you can incorporate into your Reiki Healing framework. Some of them will take a little practice but we are certain that you'll be pleased with the results. So what is the next step? Find a Mantra, pick any one that appeals to you personally or simply work through the list. If you've been keeping a progress and contemplation journal then be sure to note it as you go. You may be closer to a profound experience right now than you think so if you've got it, then keep the journal handy. Draw some excess Chi energy from your Pericardium and let's begin.

Reiki and Mantra Integration Exercises

1. Mantra: ' **Chattar Chakkar Varti**'

This is a Mantra that you can use in conjunction with Reiki Healing for anxiety. Touch your hand your skin and feel the Reiki healing energy flowing inside of you as you chant this Mantra (or mouth it silently if you're in a more public place). See the healing energy empowering your Chi to grow brighter, as light branches from the

Chi into the body to the Solar Plexus Chakra. In this way you've employed aspects of Chakra Points and the Kundalini in order to compliment the powerful Reiki healing energies. Your fear will soon be banished.

2. Mantra: **'Sa Re Sa Sa'**

This Mantra is may be used to remove negativity at the same time that it stimulates your creativity. You'll need a notebook and a pen and pencil handy (not required, necessarily, but useful for this exercise) This Mantrat associates with your Throat Chakra, so for this Reiki healing, tap your throat as you say each word of the chant and see the white light of your Chi brightening with each tap of your finger and your Throat Chakra brightening in its own blue glow. When the light of your Chi and your Throat Chakra will grow no brighter, stop tapping, and write down the first thing that comes to your mind. This will be your inspiration for a great writing or artwork, so be sure to store the notebook somewhere safe where you may consult these results as needed.

3. Mantra: **'Ra Ma Da Sa Sa Say Sohung'**

This Mantra strengthens the body and the mind, stimulating them from within as the white light of your Chi brightens and expands in harmony with this working. Best used in the morning (but you can do this any time that you wish), to use it, first place your hand, fingers spread, and touch your forehead. Focus on the repetition of the Mantra and with each repetition, see the light spreading from your forehead and down as it brightens your entire Chi. As the light goes down your body, visualize a coil of energy, your Kundalini, at the base of your spine slowly uncoiling as it rises to the Crown Chakra at the top of your head. Repeat until your Chi will grow no brighter and then go about your day confidently with your healing factors stimulated.

4. Mantra: 'Hum Dum Har Har'

This is a very powerful Mantra that can focus healing in a number of ways. It translates roughly into 'We are everything, the universe, and the Creative Infinity.'. It promotes tranquility for deep and healing rest as well as stimulating the Crown, Third Eye, and Sacral Chakra points. This allows for a more focused healing. The healing areas associated with these Chakras are as follows:

Crown Chakra

- Migraines headaches, Bipolar disorder, Thyroid issues, lack of inspiration

Third Eye Chakra

- Eye pain, insomnia, chronic headaches, loss of interest in your future

Sacral Chakra

- Bladder, back pain, Ovarian cysts, kidney problems, lack of sex drive

As you can see, there are a number of issues that may be targeted. For this healing, hold your hand open, fingers spread, and move it slowly from the Crown Chakra, down to the Third Eye, and then down to the Sacral Chakra as you chant the Mantra. Visualize light spreading from your hand and your Chi energy growing brighter as each of the three Chakras ignites in it's particular color. Violet for the Crown Chakra, Indigo for your Third Eye Chakra, and Orange for your Sacral Chakra. As your Chi blazes, move your hand to the specific Chakra area that concerns what you would like to heal. See it's light glowing as well, your Chi a circle of bright light white with the Chakra's light in the center, working in harmony. When you feel focused and centered in these energies (and you'll know) then visualize the specific area of the body that you're working to heal. See energies from your Chi and Chakra striking the area like a warm, healing lightning. Once you can visualize this and feel it's warmth, bask in it until you feel ready and then relax your breathing and open your eyes.

5. Mantra: **'Wahe Guru'**

Translating roughly into 'The ecstasy of divine wisdom that can't be described', this Mantra may be employed for lifting the spirit, strengthening the Chi, and increasing the speed at which you learn to manipulate energies. It's a Mantra of self-transformation and as such, can be one of the most healing Mantras of all. To use it, place your hand upon your face and see your Chi energy shaping brightly around you, forming an arrow pointing to the north that grows more sharply distinct with each repetition of the Mantra. Feel your mind sharpening in focus as well and think of your goal, your energies will be more aligned to the achievement of it.

6. Mantra: **'Ek ong kar sat nam siri wha hay guru'**

This Mantra is known as the 'Adi Shakti'. It translates roughly as 'In the ecstasy and bliss of Wisdom, the Creator and Creation are one'. It associates with the Solar Plexus Chakra and as such, using it with Reiki can help to focus an energy healing to the associated areas, such as the Gall Bladder, stomach, the liver, and the pancreas. To use this Mantra with a Reiki healing, hold your hand, palm open and fingers spread, over your Solar Plexus Chakra. Begin chanting the Mantra as you visualize rippling white light in your Chi with the Chakra Point glowing a brighter and brighter yellow in a solid sphere. Visualize the area that you wish to heal as well (google a picture of a healthy version of the organ that you wish to send healing energy to as an aid in your visualizations). Move your hand from the Solar Plexus Chakra to the afflicted area and see a synthesis of the White Chi and Yellow Chakra energy moving into the area.

Feel a rising heat in the area, not unpleasant, only soothing and continue the visualization and the chant for a few minutes until you feel the healing energy is well in place. Open your eyes and you're done.

7. Mantra: ' **Har Har Har Har Gobinday'**

This is a healing Mantra for the Mind, specifically for the negative results that can occur with over-contemplation of a rocky past. While it's good to learn from the past, dwelling there can cause you to trip and falter on your path to a brighter future. Use this Mantra as needed to help in dispelling the negativity so that it no longer binds you from moving forward. It associates with the Sacral Chakra which, among other things, impacts the way that we interpret the various experiences of life, be they life-affirming such as the birth of a child or deeply wounding, such as the death of someone dear.

To use this in a Reiki healing, hold your hand, palm open and fingers spread, above the Sacral Chakra. This is just below the Navel. Visualize your Chi energy flaring around you as bright white light and your Sacral Chakra responding in kind with it's deep orange light. As you chant the Mantra, see an Hourglass inside the Chakra light, full of sand at the bottom. Let the white light of your Chi energy extend inside to force it over, so that new pasts may be built on the sands of the old. Feel the old oppression losing it's hold on you. Open your eyes, confident in the knowledge that the Past is no longer everything, but rather, the steps we took to get to the steps that we now take.

8. Mantra: **'Har'**

Translated as 'The Creative Infinity', this Mantra may be utilized in Reiki healing as a means of repairing the damaged inspiration. Are you having Writer's block or trouble with an Art concept that you're developing? This Mantra can help. One of the functions of the Throat Chakra, which this Mantra associates with, is the expression of Creativity. To break the dam and let the river flow, use the following steps. First, hold your fingers close to your throat. See your Chi energy flare up as you begin the chant. The white light surrounds you and you'll let it flow like water, down from the Crown Chakra at the top of your head, past the Third Eye Chakra between above and between the brows, and finally to the Throat Chakra which will flare a bright blue. Imagine that there is an impediment here, a tiny wall which is preventing the Chi from flowing downward to the Root Chakra. Now visualize the energy pushing through violently, breaking the blockage and travelling downward through your lower Chakras. The blockage destroyed, see the Chi power travel down, like in a completed electrical circuit, until it reaches the Root Chakra. Now it travels back up, igniting each of the 7 Chakras in their colors.

Red, Orange, Yellow, Green, Blue, Indigo, and Violet..

As the Chi energy travels back up, it also moves outside of the body at the same time, creating a nimbus of light with 7 Chakra gems at the center. Enjoy the brilliance and open your eyes, it's time to express your creativity.

9. Mantra: **' Gobinde, Mukunde, Udare, Apare, Haring, Karing, Nirname, Akame'**

This Mantra translates as 'Sustainer, Liberator, Enlightener, Infinity, Destroyer, Creator, Unnamed, Without Desire'. Tied to the Heart Chakra, this Mantra can help the brain to function by lessening disharmonies. This can be used to ward off social anxiety, paranoia, false suspicions on your part, or the inability to interpret emotional responses due to disharmony of the heart and the mind. It can also be used in conjunction with your current medical regimen for irregularities of the heartbeat such as Tachycardia.

To use this Mantra with Reiki healing, hold your hand just over your Heart Chakra (your central chest) and visualize a green light growing forth organically to fill the sphere of energy of your Heart Chakra. Begin your chanting of the Mantra. See it as if the light is pulsing, in tune with your heartbeat and the individual words of the Mantra. Next, visualize your Chi energy pulsing as well, synchronized with your Heart Chakra.

If there is a particular area you wish to promote healing in, visualize it as each flash occurs. See the flashing going faster, out of synch with your heart now, until both lights of the Chi and the Heart Chakra are now a solid light and the visual of the area you wish to heal is solid, in the center of both. When you feel suffused with the healing warmth you may open your eyes, your energies are now aligned towards this healing.

10. Mantra: **"Om"**

'Om' is the sound that the Hindus believe was the first sound heard in the creation of the Universe. This Mantra can be used to heal blockages of the Throat Chakra and consequently, the areas associated with the Throat Chakra (neck, mouth, ears, the thyroid, and the Larynx). To use this Mantra with Reiki, hold your hand close to your throat, cupped, just below the chin. As you chant the Mantra, notice how it reverberates. See yourself surrounded by your Chi and pull back your vision to see the same energy surrounding you in everything. See the Throat Chakra flare up as your Chi brightens in tune with it. Continue chanting and visualize the blockage being broken or the part of the body you wish to heal glowing with a combination of both lights. Continue to pull out your view as you chant. Feel the Infinite around you before 'dropping back' to your body. Open your eyes, the working has been performed and may be repeated as needed.

11. Mantra: ' **Prana, Apana, Sushumna, Hari. Hari Har, Hari Har, Hari Har, Hari'**

'Prana' is the Hindu word for 'Life Energy', while 'Sushumna' is the 'Central Channel' through which your energies flow. Much like the Midians, actually, which is one of the reasons these systems work well together. This powerful Mantra may be used to speed up healing. To use it for a Reiki session, place your hand just in front of the center of your chest, not touching but almost touching your skin. Begin chanting the Mantra as you visualize your Chi energy moving up slowly from the base of your spine to the afflicted area.

See the area glowing with Chi light of it's own' in harmony with the Chi that surrounds your body as well as the Chi in the Universe around you. Continue the chant and the slow send of energy upwards until you feel the tingling warmth that lets you know that the energy is going where it needs to go. Now, you're done. Try this a few times a week to speed your bodie's natural healing.

12. Mantra: 'Ong Sohung'

Bearing a rough translation of 'I am the creative consciousness', this Mantra may be used in conjunction with Reiki for the healing of areas associated with the Heart Chakra (heart, breast, lungs, and upper back.). To use this, Hold your hand, palm open and fingers spread over your Heart Chakra.

Chant the Mantra in tune with the beat of your heart, one word per beat, as you visualize Chi energy flowing through your hand and filling your Heart Chakra with energy, creating a glowing green gem at the Chakra point. See the energy flowing from here to the afflicted area, infusing it with light and warmth. Do this until it seems that it can no longer contain energy and then relax your breathing and open your eyes.

13. Mantra: "Akal, Maha Kal"

With a grim translation of' Undying, Great death, this Mantra may be used with a Reiki healing to remove anxiety and fear. As we are relaxing the mind of anxiety, place your hand, palm open with fingers spread over your Solar Plexus Chakra. As you say the first sacred word, 'Akal', see the white light from your Chi flowing into your Solar Plexus Chakra and as you say the second part, 'Maha Kal' see the Chakra responding by igniting with orange fire.

Feel the fire chasing away your anxiety. Feel it burning up the fear. Repeat the Mantra and keep feeding Chi energy to empower it, until the fire of the Chi and Chakra energy has devoured all or enough of the fear and you can face things with a calm mind.

14. Mantra: '**Ad Guray Nameh, Jugad Guray Nameh, Sat Guray Nameh, Siri Guru Devay Nameh**'

Roughly translated, 'I bow to the primal teacher who takes us to the divine inspirations, I bow to the elder wisdoms, I bow to the true and hidden wisdom.'. This powerful Mantra can be used as a preventative measure from toxic personalities or as a defense from chronic anxiety. To use this in a Reiki healing (though in this case, 'preventative healing'), hold your open palm, fingers spread over each Chakra point from Root to Crown.

Visualize your Chi blazing around you, a protective white sphere of light, and begin your chant. Visualize the Chakra energies extending on both sides as you empower each, forming a crystal lattice of all of their associated colors within the circle. It may take more than one chant of the Mantra to empower each Chakra but that's okay, just do it slowly and chant as many times as you need to create the protective sphere. Once you can see it in all its glory, open your eyes and go about your day in confidence.

15. Mantra: '**Sat Narayan, Wha He Guru, Hari Narayan, Sat Nam**'

While there isn't a full translation available, Hari Narayan is essentially 'sustenance of creativity', as 'Narayan' represents the fluidity of shape that's possessed by water. This Kundalini Mantra may be used in a Reiki healing to promote clarity of thought or to promote healing. To invoke this, place an open palm on each side of your headd, fingers lightly touching the skin. Begin chanting the Mantra and see your Chi energy entering your body through your head and flowing down to the spine.

When it reaches the spine, see your Kundalini energy uncoiling from the base of your spine like a serpent and stretching slowly up to your Crown Chakra. When the energy is fully extended, let bothyour Chi and your Serpent power become brighter and brighter until their brilliance is hard to look into. Feel peaceful and safe in this glow, balanced and at one with yourself and with the Universe. This Mantra is also very good when you've just suffered a shocking or traumatic experience and wish to balance yourself by balancing your energies.

Be sure to practice your Mantras. Paste reminders on the refrigerator or on post-it notes throughout your home or work desk. There are a number of ways that you can help to remind yourself, the number one method is going to be practice, practice, practice.

We hope that you've enjoyed this new addition to your toolbox. There are more Mantras out there for you to discover, should this chapter have piqued your interest. While Mantras may serve a wide variety of purposes we wanted to provide you with the ones that fit best with our healing framework. After all, this is 'Reiki Healing for Beginners'. Next we'll add a few more tools to your tool set in a chapter entitled 'Miscellaneous Reiki Exercises'.

Chapter 10 - Reiki - Full 12 Meridian Healing

Here is a list of exercises that can help you help you in learning the Meridians. We've taken 12 exercises and turned them into one large exercise, so that you can learn and practice all 12 of the Meridians for Reiki healing. For best results, record yourself speaking so that you can play it back with music and give yourself a fully guided meditation, something that you can practice to ensure the memorization of the proper median points. Once you've learned these, combining them with the tradition based Reiki healing means that you can perform a healing that seems both simple and graceful, yet contains enough visualization and understanding of the human body in the background that it will prove effective. Don't expect to learn this overnight, it will take some time and patience, but we are certain that you'll be happy with the results. Let's now continue to the full Reiki healing so that you can learn your Meridians and go from there.

Reiki Yin and Yang Meridians - Full Healing

This is a full Reiki healing that you can perform as practice or as a form of 'preventative maintenance' to ensure that all of your Meridians are balanced. Record yourself reading it if you like and play a little music while your own voice walks you through the healing if you like. It's an excellent way to learn while encouraging good health in the body.

*Note: In this healing we are going to encompass all of your Meridians

> 1. Begin your breathing exercises. Focus on the counts of your breath until you become deeply and comfortably relaxed.
>
> 2. Place you hand, open palmed and fingers slightly spread, and place your hand just over your Heart so that you may access the Pericardium.
>
> 3. Draw Focus on your Chi. See it burning brightly around you, a white light that surrounds and fills you with joy and warmth. This same energy is in everyone and everything. It's you and it's the Universe. Take a moment to enjoy it's warmth and then we shall continue when you're ready.
>
> 4. Now that you're ready, draw excess Chi energy from your Pericardium. See it as a white light, almost to brilliant to look into, flowing into your hand, taking the form of a sphere. The first of the Yin and Yang pairings that we'll be healing are the Spleen and the Stomach. The Spleen is the Yin of this pairing, the Stomach is the Yang.

Yin and Yang 1 -The Spleen and the Stomach Meridians

> 5. Move your hand* down to your foot, placing it just over the outside edge of your big toe. This is the beginning of

your Spleen Meridian. From here, move your palm from here up the inside of your legs, seeing the ball of light getting slowly smaller as the line of the Meridian illuminates and energizes. See the Meridian brightening as the Chi sphere passes through it. Move the light up your leg and to your thigh, passing further up to your abdomen. The ball of light should be dwindled to at least three-quarters, the Meridian glowing brightly where you've already touched it with the light. Take the light up further to the outside of the nipple and up to your second rib. The light orb is smaller now, most of the Meridian glowing brightly. Now, take the light to the terminus of the Meridian, the 6th space between your ribs. Take a moment to contemplate the entire illuminated Spleen Meridian and when you're ready we shall continue.

*Note: If you're already familiar with all of the Meridians, you don't need to trace your palm over the path that the lines take, but can instead keep your hand on the Pericardium to draw forth the excess Chi and visualize the ball of energy travelling over the Meridian lines.

6. Move your hand back to your Pericardium and draw more excess Chi into your hand. Don't worry about running out... Chi is around you, inside you, and pervades the Universe and every living thing. When you've gathered the energy into a glowing white ball, let's continue and heal the Stomach Meridian.

7. Move your hand and your healing light of Chi up to your face, moving it just under the center of your eye. This is where the Meridian of your Stomach begins. Move your hand down to the very edge of your jaw, seeing the

Meridian line brighting as you pass the light through it. Move your open palm slowly down your throat, almost touching but not quite, as the glowing orb feeds the Meridian and grows slowly smaller, continuing down to your abdomen and further down across the front of your leg.

Move the ball of light, now just a fraction of it's previous size, all the way down to your foot where the last of the light is absorbed at the terminus of the Meridian, the nail of your second toe. Take a moment to see the Meridian in its entirety, glowing brightly from the excess Chi that you've pushed there to imbalance and clear it of blockage. Once you've contemplated the Stomach Meridian then we can move on to the next pairing.

8. Move your hand, palm open and fingers lightly spread so that it's place over your Pericardium. Gather energy as before from your excess Chi, willing it into the shape of a ball of light hovering beneath your palm. We'll now 'trace' and heal the next two Meridians.

Yin and Yang 2 - The Lungs and The Large Intestine Meridians

9. Now we are going to heal the Yin of this pairing, the Lungs. Move your hand up close to your shoulder to the first space between your ribs. This is called the intercostal space and it's the starting point of the Lung Meridian. See the Meridian line flaring up as you pass the orb over it.

Move it up to the shoulder and down the front of your arm, the energy slowly transferring from the sphere of light in your palm as the Meridian is energized, dwindling to nothing as you take it down to the terminus of this Meridian, the fingernail of your thumb. Take a moment to admire the Lung Meridian, blazing brightly to your heightened senses. When you're ready, let's continue.

10. Move your hand back to your Pericardium and draw more excess Chi into your hand.

11. The Yang of the pairing is the Meridian of your Large Intestine. Move your open palm to your opposite hand to the beginning of this Meridian, the fingernail of your index finger. See the line shining as you direct the Chi energy in your hand to it and bring the light up your arm, tothe back of your shoulder, the ball of light becoming smaller as it's energy expends to balance and unblock this Meridian.

From the back of your shoulder, bring your hand up to your face to the terminus of this Meridian, your nostrils. Take a moment to observe the shining trail that the Large Intestine Meridian travels through your body and commit it to memory. When you're ready to continue we can go on to the next step.

12. Move your hand back to your Pericardium and draw more excess Chi into your hand.

Yin and Yang 3 - The Liver and the Gall Bladder Meridians

13. The Yin of our next pairing is the Liver. Move your open palm down to your foot and to our large toe. The Meridian begins just under the nail. See it lighten up with crackling, white Chi energy as you bring the orb to it's beginning. Move the orb in your hand slowly up your inner leg, moving next to your thigh.

See the energy dwindling, the orb shrinking slowly as you move along, the Meridian growing brighter as you pass. From the thigh, bring the light up the outside of your abdomen to it's terminus, your Sternum. Admire the newly illuminated path of the Liver Meridian for a moment to better commit it to memory and when you're ready, let's continue.

14. Move your hand back to your Pericardium and draw more excess Chi light into your hand.

15. The Yang of this pairing is the Gall Bladder. Let's heal this Meridian now. Move your hand up your face to the starting point of this Meridian, the outer corner of your eye. Visualize the start of the Meridian line flaring up as it greets the energy you're putting into it and will the Chi orb inside of your head and downward, where your hand will meet it at the front of your shoulder.

From here pass it down to your abdomen, noting how the orb is slowly dwindling as the Meridian grows brighter where it has been touched. Keep moving your hand down but release the orb to go inside of your abdomen, when it goes further down the Meridian at the bottom of your abdomen. Take the orb down the outer side of your leg to your foot and the Meridian's terminus, the nail or your fourth toe. Take a moment of contemplation to commit it to memory and then we shall move on. to the next pairing.

16. Move your hand once more to your Pericardium and collect more Chi energy.

Yin and Yang 4 - The Kidneys and the Bladder Meridians

17. The Yin of this pairing is the Kidneys Meridian. Move your hand down to the sole of your foot where this Meridian begins. See the Meridian flaring to life as you release some of the Chi energy into it. Move the Chi orb up the inside of your leg, noting as it slowly gets smaller and the Meridian brightens.

From the inside of your leg, move the light upwards to your abdomen and up further still to the terminus of this Meridian, the Clavicle. Take a moment to observe the brightened and empowered Meridian and commit it's path to memory and then we shall continue.

17. Collect more Chi energy from your Pericardium.

18. The Yang of this pairing is your Bladder. Move your Chi orb up to your face to the start of this Meridian, the inner-corner of your eye. Move the light over the top of your head and down your back (if not limber, you can visualize the orb moving by itself down your back). See it dwindling as it expends power slowly, causing the Meridian to crackle with energy as you move it further still, down your leg, li

Kidneys (Yin) and Bladder (Yang)

Bladder: This Meridian starts at the inner corner of your eye, where it then goes over the top of your head, moving down your back and leg until it terminates at the toenail of your pinky (smallest toe), absorbing the orb completely at last and leaving behind it a glowing trail that's your Bladder Meridian.

Take a moment to appreciate this line of power that the Ancients hold in such esteem. Commit to memory what you can and let's continue with the next pairing after charging up.

19. Gather a ball of healing energy from your Pericardium.

Yin and Yang 5 - The Heart and the Small Intestine

20. The Yin of this pairing is the Heart Meridian. It starts in your arm pit, so move your hand there and ignite the Meridian with the Chi energy that you've gathered in your hand. See it flaring up in response and bring the light further along the Meridian, down your inner arm and to your hand as the ball quickly dwindles and feeds energy into this shining line until finally expending itself at the terminus, your smallest finger. Take a moment to admire and memorize this simple, yet oh-so-important Meridian.

21. Move your hand over your Pericardium, palm-open and fingers outstretched slightly as you collect more excess Chi for the next step.

22. The Yang of this pairing is your Small Intestine Meridian. To begin, move your empowered hand to your opposite hand, placing it over the beginning of this Meridian, your smallest finger. See the Meridian brightening as you activate it like a circuit with your Chi energy.

Move your hand up the Meridian by taking it along the back of your arm, watching the energy dwindle slowly as you bring it up to your shoulder. Watch the orb, growing smaller as the Meridian grows brighter while you bring it down the shoulder, then up to your neck, finally moving it to its terminus, your ear, where it swallows the last of the energy. Take a moment to commit the path of this Meridian to memory and then we are ready to continue to the last pairing.

23. Move your hand to the Pericardium, with your palm open and held barely above the spot. Pull the excess Chi energy and shape it into a ball of healing white light.

Yin and Yang 6 - The Pericardium and the Triple Warmer

24. The Pericardium is the Yin of this pairing. Move your hand to the outside of the nipple in order to touch the Chi light to this location, as it's the beginning of this Meridian. See the Meridian responding to the energy that the orb provides it.

From here, move the orb up your shoulder, seeing it becoming slightly smaller as the Meridian becomes *brighter and you pass it down the front of your arm and to your hand. See the orb of light, tiny now. become absorbed as you reach the Meridian's terminus, your middle-finger. See the Meridian, bright and shining now and note the path for when you need it next time.*

25. Gather up more excess Chi from your newly cleansed and empowered Pericardium, shaping the energy into a ball for the last portion of our healing.

26. The Triple Warmer is the Yang of this pairing and it's fitting that we do this last. As we've mentioned, this Meridian is important in that it governs your metabolism, body heat, and distribution of liquids throughout the entire body. After any healing is done this Meridian should be healed as well in case of imbalance or blockage from the Meridian that was blocked.

To heal this Meridian, move your open palm over the nail of your ring finger. See the Meridian respond, flaring to life as you bring the healing light up your forearm and continue up, the light sphere slowly growing smaller as the Meridian grows brighter as you move it to the back of your shoulder. From here, bring the light up to your ear and let its remaining energy all be absorbed at the terminus of this Meridian, your eyebrow.

27. Take a moment to contemplate the Triple Warmer Meridian, as well as all of the others which we've worked with in this healing.

Do you have all of the Meridians committed to memory yet? Keep practicing and soon you'll know them by heart. Good job, and consider this healing a success!

You've learned the Meridians. We can only give you the wisdom and knowledge. what you do with it's up to you. Take some time, let it soak in, learn every pathway, know your body, know your mind, know what the ancients wanted you to know. A system so old, you should take in the best of it and improve your understanding. Take the path of wisdom. You've come this far, why not go farther?

Chapter 11 - Healing stones to incorporate into Reiki and Chakra Healings

The following is a list of stones in the colors of your 7 Chakra points. These can be incorporated into healings by the placement of the appropriate color stones on its corresponding Chakra point before beginning the Reiki healing. Procure one or many of each color to add their natural influences while you're stimulating the Chakras and ensuring a more patient-specific healing session when you're performing Reiki. If needed, feel free to loan out stones with specific properties after a healing or acquire extra for distribution to patients. The results from adding these stones to your healings can be quite satisfying.

Red Stones

1. Rhodonite

Healing Properties: Possessed of a lovely rose hue, this stone is famous for its properties in emotional healing. This is one that you'll definitely want to add to your collection. This silicate is good for calming anger and for the healing of traumas as well. Find it, add it to your healing toolbox.

2. Rose Quartz

Healing Properties: A powerful healer of the Heart both spiritually and physically, Rose Quartz can help you to open yourself emotionally when you've been wounded in the past. It also promotes a healthy circulatory system and strengthens your

Heart. It's also very easy to obtain a nice piece for yourself, so be sure to add this to your collection soon.

3. Ruby

Healing Properties: Revered long by the ancients, legend has it that Kublai Khan once offered a city in exchange for a sizeable and apparently quite exquisite specimen. Thankfully in this day and age, you can obtain your own Ruby for quite a bit less (especially if purchased raw). Ruby inspires a vigor of the spirit and the body, driving one to live more fully. It can also assist with sexual dysfunction, fever, and constriction of the blood vessels. Star Ruby is said to have the same healing qualities, but magnified.

4. Bloodstone

Healing Properties: Bloodstone is good for detoxification and grounding negative energy. In matters of the heart it can help to ground negativity as well so this is a good stone to keep close.

5. Garnet

Healing Properties: Known as a simulator of creativity, Garnet is also a stone of sensuality, inciting passion into your love life and keepings things fresh.

6. Red Coral

Healing Properties: Strengthening circulation, as well as healing of the kidneys and the bladder, this stone pushes even further and assists in overall regeneration. The stone that grows like a plant can serve you well. Red Coral also acts as a natural antidepressant, so consider it for your healing toolbox.

Orange Stones

1. Spessartine Garnet

Healing Properties: Sometimes called 'the Garnet of the Sun', Spessartine Garnet can boost creativity as well as enhance cognitive function in matters of logic. This is a good stone to have when you're looking to make a life change as well, as the stone's energies are well aligned in that regard.

2. Orange Sunstone

Healing Properties: Nurturing feelings of generosity, the Orange Sunstone also empowers those who have lost a loved one with needed strength to weather the seperation and move on. This stone also has a balancing and cleansing effect on all of the Chakras. This is also an excellent stone to have for empowering yourself against phobias through its joyful nature.

3. Carnelian

Healing Properties: Good for arthritis, lower back problems, and issues with the kidneys, Carnelian is also a good stone to have for stabilizing in the wake of an abusive relationship. It promotes accelerated healing and is also good for dealing with depression.

4. Orange Agate

Healing Properties: Orange Agate is an emotional stabilizer. Helping to keep you grounded, this is a good stone for anger management as well as for avoiding impulse decisions.

5. Orange Sapphire

Healing Properties: Orange Sapphire is a good stone for Artists and Writers, inspiring creativity. Use this to dispel writer's block or other issues of stifled creativity.

6. Orange Citrine

Healing Properties: Orange citrine is a promotes cognition. Physically, it helps to cleanse the kidneys, aids in digestion, detoxifies the blood and balances the thyroid. This is another good addition to your collection.

7. Amber

Healing Properties: Aiding in physical regeneration, Amber also acts as a natural purifier. Good for chronic pain, Amber also has a cleansing effect on all of the Chakra points. Amber is also reputed to draw sickness and disease from the body as well, due to its purification properties

8. Hessonite Garnet

Healing Properties: Hessonite Garnet is a powerful stone for treating ailments of the mind. Providing clarity of thought and confidence in the face of one's fears.

Yellow Stones

1. Iron Pyrite (also called Fool's Gold)

Healing Properties: Acting as a powerful shield from negative energies, Iron Pyrite also enhances memory and is good for the healing of bones, reduction in swelling, and conditions of the lungs.

2. Yellow Citrine

Healing Properties: Good for anxiety, Yellow Citrine also acts as an amplifier for energies. This stone also aids in the treatment of eye issues as well, which empowering your lower 3 Chakras and your Third Eye Chakra as well.

3. Canary Yellow Tourmaline

Healing Properties: Canary Yellow Tourmaline works as a powerful mental stabilizer, as such it's good for anxiety, phobias, and can even help with Bipolar disorder. This stone can balance all of the Chakras as well so it's a good one to have around for your collection.

4. Gold

Healing Properties: Gold is good for a number of healing applications. For one, it acts as a natural amplifier to any minerals that it's paired with. Healing-wise, gold is said to help with issues such as the treatment of the nervous system, breathing issues, rejuvenation of the endocrine system and regeneration of tissue.

5. Lemon Quartz

Healing Properties: Lemon Quartz has a number of uses, including resistance to food and nicotine cravings, faster recovery following surgery, and promoting clarity of thought.

6. Yellow Sapphire

Healing Properties: Yellow Sapphires healing qualities tend more towards the spiritual, as it encourages one to turn creativity into action. As such it can be used to inspire and break through creative blocks or other hindrances in life.

7. Crysoberyl

Healing Properties: Crysoberyl is good for healing of chest and liver issues. It's also good for skin problems, digestion issues, balancing the adrenal glands, and has a positive effect regarding the balance of cholesterol in your body.

8. Golden Beryl

Healing Properties: Opening the Purple and Yellow Chakras, Golden Beryl is good for achieving a calm and peaceful state of emotions. This is a good stone to have when recovering from mental trauma as it can help to soothe the weary spirit.

Green Stones

1. Green Aventurine

Healing Properties: Good for the lungs, heart, the sinuses, and the liver, this is an excellent stone to include in an intensive healing session. This stone is also said to enhance creativity.

2. Chrysoprase

Healing Properties: Stimulating your Orange and Green Chakras, Chrysoprase healing your inner child or a broken heart. Phsycially, it acts as a strong detoxifier for the liver and combats insomnia for a restful and good nights sleep.

3. Serpentine

Healing Properties: An excellent stone to include in Reiki healings, Serpentine assists in the directing of healing energies. Another detoxifier, Serpentine can help in cleansing toxins from your body and also helps in treating hypoglycemia.

4. Hiddenite

Healing Properties: This stone is good for deep emotional healing, such as for victims of abuse, addition, or those in the severe throes of grief for a lost loved one.

5. Jade

Healing Properties: Jade is good for conditions of the Spleen, the Kidneys, and the Bladder. It also boosts mental access to the spiritual world and inspires creativity.

6. Peridot

Healing Properties: Revered by Egyptian kings to the extent that touching one without permission was grounds for death, the Peridot is good for treating tobacco and other addictions. Especially prized for Reiki healing, the Peridot can help in guiding your hands as well as for recovery of energies after healings.

7. Chalcedony

Healing Properties: Good for the healing of bones, your circulatory system, eyes, and your spleen, Chalcedony is a good multifunction healer to add to your collection of healing stones.

8. Green Agate

Healing Properties: Green agate is primarily used for bringing the body and mind back into harmony. Emotionally it's good for dealing with repressed anger and fears, due to the calming influence exerted by the stone.

9. Green Garnet

Healing Properties: Encouraging regeneration and growth, this stone also increases vitality and promotes an air of compassion when dealing with others.

10. Amazonite

Healing Properties: Amazonite enhances communication, imparting the ability to see things from the point of view of others. This stone is good for healing creative blocks and for opening the closed mind.

11. Green Apatite

Healing Properties: Enhancing hand and eye coordination, Green Apatite is useful for healing in that it helps to maintain a good and stable energy flow at the same time that it's stimulating your Green Chakra.

12. Emerald

Healing Properties: Emerald is good for invigorating thought and useful in the treatment of a damaged memory. It's also good for reviving passions in one who has suffered from abuse or addiction and is seeking to enjoy life anew.

Blue Stones

1. Aquamarine

Healing Properties: Good for hormonal issues, throat problems, Thyroid issues, and swollen glands, Aquamarine is a good stone to have in your healing collection.

2. Labradorite

Healing Properties: Good for detoxification from alcohol or tobacco, this stone also helps to stabilize more negative aspects of our personalities, such as anger, envy, jealousy, and such.

3. Blue Lace Agate

Healing Properties: This stone opens and clears the Throat Chakra, as well as promoting energies that help you to destroy old patterns and modes of thinking that have proven destructive in your current life.

4. Aragonite

Healing Properties: Stimulating the Green, Blue, and Indigo Chakras, this stone promotes communication and healing from past traumas. It also amplifies empathy, which can prove quite useful for healers.

5. Blue Apatite

Healing Properties: A creativity enhancer, this stone also promotes hunger suppression so it can be useful for those trying to lose weight.

6. Celestine

Healing Properties: Another creativity stimulator, this stone is also good for dispelling anxiety. It's also attuned to the celestial and can increase the strength of guidance for the hand positions employed in Reiki healings.

7. Benetoite

Healing Properties: A stimulator of the Indigo Chakra, this stone is good for lethargy, imparting energy to get through the day for those who find themselves always tired.

8. Azurite

Healing Properties: Azurite is a stone that stimulates all of the mind, making it a good healer for those who are feeling burnt-out or who find themselves stuck in a cycle of despair.

9. Blue Topaz

Healing Properties: Stimulating the Indigo Chakra as well as the Blue Chakra, this stone can help to heal phobias associated with public speaking, boosting confidence and communication abilities.

10. Blue Aventurine

Healing Properties: This is a stone that asserts willpower for overcoming negative habits. Use it for assistance in quitting smoking, overcoming anger, substance abuse, and more. This stone can impart that additional 'oomph.' that you need to get the job done.

11. Turquoise

Healing Properties: Considered sacred by the Native Americans and other cultures, such as the Tibetans and early Egyptians, this stone has a number of properties. Good for the immune system, your bones, and for detoxifying the body, this stone also assists in effective communication with others.

12. Blue Sapphire

Healing Properties: Another stone that grants guidance of the hands, this stone is popular with Reiki healers. A stone of love, Sapphire can impart understanding of higher ideals and help to suppress feelings of powerlessness and break blocks from a focus that has been reduced to the micro level from extreme traumas in life.

Indigo Stones

1. Indigo Crystal

Healing Properties: Indigo crystals are the perfect stone for focusing self examination, a detachment of thought that explores the possibilities as envisioned from the minds of others. Use these in healing someone who clings too hard to ego. If they're sensitive, then advise that it's a stone for empathy, not all are ready to divorce their ego for truth.

2. Indigo Labradorite

Healing Properties: This stone assists with disorders of the mind and of the eyes. This stone works with the Triple Warmer, regulating metabolism and hormones. Keep this stone handy for imparting power in the closing healings of your Reiki sessions.

3. Iolite

Healing Properties: A motivator, Iolite restores perspective. This is a strong stone to incorporate into healings where there are issues with one's family.

4. Tanzanite

Healing Properties: Strengthening te Indigo Chakra, this stone can assist in empowering intuition. This stone is best used when fueling a burnt-out sense of spirituality.

5. Crystal Sodalite

Healing Properties: Assisting with calcium deficiencies, this stone can also quicken the immune system, as well as functioning as a metabolism booster. A good stone to have handy.

Violet Stones

1. Violet Sodalite

Healing Properties: Encouraging rational though, Violet sodalite also helps in preventing panic attacks.

2. Amethyst

Healing Properties :Inducing calm, this stone is paramount in matters of the nervous system. This stone is also strong in strengthening relationships.

3. Violet Topaz

Healing Properties: Recharges all of the Meridians and aids in spiritual insight.

4. Violet Beryl

Healing Properties: Provides a magnification effect to healings, this is a must-have for the more serious practitioners.

5. Violet Tourmaline

Healing Properties: Reducing fear, this stone breaks creativity blocks and pushes overall happiness.

6. Jadeite

Healing Properties: Protecting against fatigue, enhancing the circulatory system, and empowering longevity, think of this as the 'long life' stone.

7. Spinel

Healing Properties: Revitalization in the face of challenges, this stone helps the recipient to deal with problems as they would in youth and power. Providing a fount of seemingly endless energy, this is the stone for te conquering of will over want.

8. Violet apatite

Healing Properties: Enhancing the Blue Chakra, this stone sharpens communication to a level tat is almost the poet. Use sparingly, sometimes people react poorly to the world described with accuracy, especially the personal world.

9. Barite

Healing Properties: Energy alignment and spiritual focus, this is for those who are ready to progress.

Conclusion

You've learned about Meridians, standard Reiki, and gone well on your path for healing others and self-healing. We've gone into Mantras and Chakra points, in order to ensure that you not only have the basics, but that you're educated in what you need to know to get started effectively.

Be sure to practice the Meridians, learn the Traditional hand placements, and then take that knowledge and build from there. Once you've done the healing exercises a number of times and once you've seen the results then we are certain that you'll be happy with the fruits of your labor.

Now you've started you Reiki journey, you'll find it will lead you to new insights, discoveries, body-mind healing techniques, and even new people and places. Reiki is spreading rapidly around the world and we are constantly learning more about it's profound healing capabilities, so make sure you continue to practice and deepen your knowledge in this wonderful ancient art of healing.

Peace and blessings to you all,

Siya Ishani

www.ingramcontent.com/pod-product-compliance
Lightning Source LLC
Chambersburg PA
CBHW071958070526
44583CB00015B/1248